Vegan Meal Prep

Easy, Delicious, and Healthy Plant Based Meals, Snacks, Shopping Lists, and Meal Plans That Save You Time and Money (Healthy Eating Made Simple)

Table of Contents

Introduction 4
Chapter 1: What is Veganism? 7
Chapter 2: Your Guide to Vegan Nutrition ... 22
Chapter 3: Are There Any Deficiencies to Worry About? 43
Chapter 4: Everything You Need to Know About Meal Planning 48
Chapter 5: Nutrient Dense Vegan Foods to Get Started 61
Chapter 6: How to Store Your Food 66
Chapter 7: Staples In Every Vegans Kitchen . 80
Chapter 8: Week One Meal Plan and Grocery List 91
Chapter 9: Week Two Meal Plan and Grocery List 136
Chapter10: Week Three Meal Plan and Grocery List 183
Chapter 11: Week Four Meal Plan and Grocery List 213
Chapter 12: Week Five Meal Plan and Grocery List 240

Chapter 13: Week Six Meal Plan and Grocery List 268

Conclusion 293

Introduction

Congratulations on downloading *Vegan Meal Prep* and thank you for doing so.

The following chapters will discuss everything that you need to know in order to get started with the vegan diet and to ensure that you learn the basics that come with meal prepping. Going on a vegan diet can be tough, and making sure that you have the right foods and meals ready ahead of time when you are starting with a new diet plan, and when you are busy and tired, can be hard. But when you meal plan along with the vegan diet, things are going to be so much easier and you will love the results.

This guidebook is going to spend some time looking at both the vegan diet plan and some of the basics that you are able to work with when you are trying to meal plan. When you combine both, you are going to see some amazing results, without all of the hassle and without feeling stressed out.

This guidebook is going to start out with what you need to know in order to get started with the vegan diet. We will talk about what the vegan diet is, some of the reasons that people choose to go on a vegan diet, the importance of getting the right nutrition, and how to avoid any deficiencies that can come up.

From there, we will move on to some of the things that you need to know about meal planning on this diet plan. There are so many benefits that can come from being on a meal plan, whether you are doing the vegan diet or not. And learning how to do it in the proper way can make all of the difference. Here, we will look at the benefits of meal planning, how to keep the right foods in your pantry, how to store foods properly and more.

The final section of this guidebook is going to be your favorite part when you first get started with meal planning on the vegan diet. It contains a meal plan, recipes, and a shopping list for your first six weeks on this plan. No more scrounging around for the information you need. No more hours spent online or in cookbooks trying to think of ideas.It is all presented to you here in this guidebook, to make things so much easier overall.

When you are ready to get started on the vegan diet and want to add in some meal planning to make your life easier, check out this guidebook to learn how you can get all this done!

There are plenty of books on this subject on the market, therefore, thanks again for choosing this one. Every effort was made to ensure it is full of as much useful information as possible, so please enjoy!

Chapter 1: What is Veganism?

The first question that a lot of readers are going to ask is "what is veganism?" If you are coming here looking for a brand new way to take care of yourself and to ensure that you are able to eat healthy and nutritious foods, rather than filling your body with junk food that is not good for you at all, then veganism is a great place to start. But before we get started, we need to have an idea of what veganism is all about.

To make this simple, veganism is any abstinence from the use of animal products. This is both in the diet and in the lifestyle of the individual who follows it. It is slightly different from vegetarianism, so it is important to keep these two separate. Vegetarianism still allows you to eat some animal products like milk, eggs, and cheese, but veganism requires that you abstain from these products.

In addition to being careful about the types of foods that you eat on this diet plan, those on the vegan diet are also careful about the products they use. You will not find these individuals wearing anything made of leather, for example. They are worried about the treatment of animals, don't like that animals are being abused, and other reasons that prevent them from eating or wearing animal products.

A great explanation of ethical veganism comes from a group known as the International Vegetarian Union. According to them, "Veganism may be defined as a way of living that seeks to exclude, as far as possible and practical, all forms of exploitation of, and cruelty to, animals for food, clothing, or for any other purpose. In dietary terms, it refers to the practice of dispensing with all animal products, including meat, fish, poultry, animal milk, honey, and their derivatives.

As you can see, there are some restrictions on the kinds of foods that you are allowed to eat on this plan. But if you are worried about how animals are being exploited in our modern world, and you want to take care of your health in the process, then veganism is the right choice for you.

Why do people adopt the vegan lifestyle?

There are many reasons why someone may choose to adopt this kind of lifestyle. Some of the most common reasons that you will hear in favor of the vegan lifestyle include:

1. Issues of animal welfare and the objection of seeing and using any kind of animal as a commodity.
2. Issues with the environment that are directly tied back with animal agriculture. These can be things like

contaminated drainage from farms and air pollution. These individuals may choose to become vegan in order to lessen over-consumption of resources including fossil fuels, water, and land.

3. By adopting veganism, these individuals may see it as a part of the solution to world hunger because they are being more efficient in the way they utilize the resources of this world.

4. There are some vegans who are known as dietary vegans. These individuals choose to follow a plant-based diet because they want to help improve their health overall. They may not choose to avoid other animal products in their life, and will just follow this with their dietary choices.

What can I eat as a vegan?

When you first hear about the vegan diet, you may feel like there are just so many different foods that have to be cut out of the mix. You may worry that this is going to be too hard to keep up with. Because we are so used to eating whatever we want, it can seem a bit hard to imagine that we need to cut down on a full food group, and sometimes more than one.

But as you start to look more at the vegan diet, and some of the recipes that we will show in this guidebook, it won't take long to see that there are actually a lot of different foods that you can eat and still maintain this diet plan. Some of the options that are available to those who decide to go on the vegan diet will include

1. Every type of fruit
2. Every type of vegetable

3. Nuts and seeds are allowed on this diet
4. You can enjoy plenty of healthy carbs. It is best to go with whole wheat options.
5. Beans and legumes are good as well.
6. Non-dairy milk such as soy milk and almond milk.
7. Chocolate. Many varieties of dark chocolate and other non-dairy milk chocolates that are out there.

What do I need to exclude when I am living as a vegan?

To keep it simple, all types of animal products are going to be avoided when you are on a vegan diet. This is going to include options like honey, eggs, dairy, seafood, poultry, meat, and any of their byproducts.

In addition to these products, the lifestyle of a vegan is going to include having to avoid animal products that show up in our day to day life as well. This can include, but is not limited to:

1. Products that the company decided to test on animals.
2. Fabrics that are derived from animals, including wool and silk.
3. All fur, down suede, and leather.
4. Any kind of personal care product that includes ingredients from animals. This would include ingredients like lanolin, keratin, and beeswax.
5. Animals that are used as entertainment, such as those in rodeos and circuses.

Of course, you can see that it is almost impossible to avoid all of the animal products out there, but this is why the International Vegetarian Union talks about how you should exclude these products "as far as possible and practical." If it isn't possible to do so, then it is fine to use something that has an animal product or byproduct in it.

Following the guidelines that are given for a vegan diet can seem difficult when you first get started. This is especially true when you are a big fan of meat and animal products. But learning how to cut some of these things out can help to protect animals, protect the environment, and help you to stay healthy and lose weight, all at the same time.

The main reasons to become Vegan

Another worry that a lot of people have when they first consider becoming vegan is why they should do it. Are they really going to be able to make that big of an impact on the world around them by eating meat and animal products along the way? Is what they do really enough to make any difference? There are a lot of reasons that people choose to go on a vegan diet, and understanding how each of these works, and how each vegan is completely different, can make the experience that much better.

The first reason to become a vegan is that eating meat is not really necessary. While there are diet plans out there that swear up and down that you must have meat, there is no proof that you need to eat the flesh of an animal or any animal by-products in order to be healthy. There are actually some studies that talk about how it is best not to eat meat at all, which is what the vegan diet promotes.

The next benefit is that being vegan is one of the healthiest diet plans out there that you can follow. Without touching on the fact that many animals are on antibiotics and hormones that can be passed on to you and are really bad, there are a ton of other health reasons why you would want to choose the vegan diet. These will include:

1. Being vegan can help to reduce your chances of developing cancer. Many meat products, especially the kinds that are processed, contain the same cancer-causing agents as cigarettes.
2. Being vegan is going to be so good for your heart.
3. Being vegan is going to help you to lower your cholesterol levels automatically. Since animal products are the only ones that contain cholesterol, and you are cutting these out, you get the benefit of not having to deal with this.
4. Vegans who follow the diet well, often have a reduced risk of gallstones, cancers, large bowel disorders, high blood pressure, coronary heart disease, and obesity. Being vegan is also going to help reduce coronary artery disease and strokes.

5. Being vegan can help prevent food poisoning since most of these cases are linked to animal products.
6. Your bowels are going to be able to work much better than before, which can do wonders when it comes to keeping the whole system healthy.
7. In one 21-year long study, it was shown that the higher the consumption of meat, the greater the death rate from all of the causes combined. This means that being vegan can help you live longer.

Being a vegan also means that you are willing to protect the planet and our world for future generations. You can go on this diet by saving trees and reducing the amount of forest that is destroyed and used for cow pastures. Between the years 1960 and 1985 alone, almost 40 percent of all the rain forests in Central America were destroyed in order to create grazing land for cows, the same ones served in

Europe and North America later on. When you go vegan, you are able to save at least one acre of rain forest each year.

Being a vegan means that you use less water. It is estimated that more than half of the water used in the United States is used to raise and kill the animals that we eat. If you stop eating animals, less water is going to be used.

Many vegans are proud of how they are able to help limit the amount of fossil fuels that are used. Just to produce one hamburger, you will use up enough fossil fuel to drive a small car, 20 miles. And since you are using up less fossil fuel, you are also creating less pollution. Animal feces and their gasses are known to be a big contributor to global warming and acid rain. Plus they pollute watersheds and rivers constantly.

Another benefit is that being vegan allows you to consider the welfare of humans as a whole. We are able to feed more people in the world on the food that animals, raised as food, eat. The amount of vegetable protein that has been used to feed a whole herd of beef in the United States would be able to feed the entire population of China and India, which is almost two billion people.

With this in mind, it is possible to make some changes in the priorities we have when it comes to eating meat and animal products, and we could end world hunger. We already have all of the resources to do it, except for our lust for eating flesh. When you go on a vegan diet, you are able to cut out some of this waste and do something that can benefit the welfare of humanity.

Many people believe that following a vegan diet is one of the most compassionate ways to exist in our world. Animals feel pain just like the rest of us. There is no argument about this. So why would someone choose to torture something just to make themselves feel good? You are able to show that you are a caring person when you go on a vegan diet.

Modern agriculture seeks to keep all animals, including ducks, turkeys, chickens, pigs, calves, and cows, in overcrowded sheds, cages, crates, and stalls, ones that are so small that they are not even able to turn around. Here, they are deprived of movement, sunlight, and even care from a vet. And eating meat allows these farmers and those concerned to take advantage of the animals around them.

When you decide to stop eating meat and animal products, you will not have to worry about this happening as much. And the more people you can influence to follow this kind of diet plan, the easier it is for you to put an end to this tragic treatment on animals. Veganism can help you to have a clear conscience and avoid forcing pain to anything that is sentient.

Even if you are not concerned about the treatment of animals, but let's be real, we all are and we can feel good knowing that veganism can help these animals, going vegan can help save you money. Nutrition from plants is going to cost a lot less than the nutrition that you get from animals. Think about it, when you need to feed a lot of people for less money, do you go out and purchase a big steak, or do you purchase some rice and beans? Plus, these plant-based foods are going to taste great and you are going to feel amazing, all at the same time.

There are a lot of reasons why one would choose to go on a vegan diet. This diet plan can help you to lose weight and protect the environment, keep animals safe, end world hunger, and promote a safer world for all of us. No matter what your reasons are for going on the vegan diet and there are so many to choose from, your life is going to improve in no time.

Chapter 2: Your Guide to Vegan Nutrition

When you go on a vegan diet, you may be worried about how you are going to be able to take care of your nutrition, and how you will be able to ensure that you eat enough vitamins and minerals to be healthy. Since we are worried about missing out on full food groups without protein, eggs, and dairy products, this is a valid concern.

It is possible to go through and work with a vegan diet and eat a bunch of junk. Technically, a lot of the junk and processed foods that are out there are bad for your body. You have to make sure that you are following the vegan diet in the proper manner so that you get the full benefits that come with this kind of diet plan. If you decide to follow the vegan diet and eat a bunch of baked goods, you are going to ruin your health and run into issues with vegan nutrition. But if you choose to eat lots of healthy fruits and vegetables, and other healthy ingredients like we will talk about in this guidebook, you will never have to worry about nutrition because you will be eating just what your body needs.

There are a number of things that you are able to do to make sure that you are getting the proper nutrition on a regular basis while on this diet plan. Some of the best ways to ensure that you are able to get some nutrition, and feel amazing, even when you cut out the meat and animal products that you are used to enjoying include:

Eat more of the plants

There are going to be a few nutrient concerns when you first start on this diet because you are avoiding animal products. But these are more so about not eating enough plants rather than not eating animals. The issues that you are going to run into are going to be because you aren't eating enough of the healthy produce that your body needs, rather than because you are missing out on animal products.

The Academy of Nutrition and Dietetics states that an appropriately planned out vegan diet is going to be healthy, no matter what stage of life you are in. This same group also advices that these plant-based diets can help to provide you with a lot of great health benefits, as long as they are done in the right way. Of course, a vegan diet that is not planned out properly could end up being dangerous. But this is the same kind of thing that you will find when you are dealing with an omnivore who isn't on this kind of diet.

It is all about making sure that you eat the right kinds of foods. If you go on a vegan diet and don't eat the right kinds of foods, you are not going to get the benefits. This is where meal planning comes into play. You will be able to follow this diet and use it in order to make sure that you are taking in the right kind of nutrition along the way.

A well-planned vegan diet is key.

Although you will find that a vegan diet is healthy no matter what stage of life you are in, it is so important that you add in some planning to make sure that you are able to get what you need out of it. In the beginning, as you are adjusting to the diet plan and learning what you are able to consume and what to avoid, you may find that working with some supplementation is needed. In addition, you need to make an effort to eat the right foods, do some self-monitoring, and be aware of your health to make sure that you are doing this properly.

If you are going on the vegan diet and you plan to stay with this kind of diet for the long term, and not just for short term weight loss, then you need to take the right measures in order to ensure that you don't miss any nutrients that are vital. It is hard to make sure that you are getting the nutrients that you need if you don't take the time to plan things out ahead of time.

The recipes that we provide in this guidebook are going to make this a whole lot easier. We have a lot of great recipes that you can use for six weeks in order to ensure that you are getting the right nutrients that your body needs. With a six-week plan, you are going to be set to eat healthy and stay on this vegan diet, without feeling like you are missing out when you eat these meals.

How much do I need to eat?

This is an area that a lot of people are going to get mixed up in. Some will eat too little on the diet plan, and some are going to eat too much when they first get started. You need to make sure that you are taking in enough calories so that your body gets the micronutrients, protein, fats, and carbs that are needed to maintain your health.

While this diet does allow a lot of fruits and vegetables to keep you healthy and help you get adequate amounts of nutrition, you will find that they are really low in calories. And aside from starchy vegetables, such as those found in potatoes, you are going to need to eat large amounts of these to get enough calories in the day.

While you should definitely make sure that you are eating plenty of fruits and vegetables when you are on this diet plan, or you aren't going to feel that good, this isn't the only thing that you need to eat each day. Whole grains and legumes are denser and will provide you with more calories and fats. These can add up quickly and will help you fill in some of the gaps that fruits and vegetables, although really good for you, just won't be able to do.

When you are planning out your diet on the vegan meal plan, a good portion of your calories need to come with carbs along with some fats and protein to help you to get everything that your body needs. Adding in some legumes, some carbs, and lots of fruits and vegetables can help you to do this.

The nutrients you need

In addition to some of the nutrients that we talked about above (mainly the Macronutrients of fat, protein, and carbs) there are a lot of different micronutrients that your body needs to help you stay as healthy as possible. Missing out on these, whether you are on the vegan diet or another diet plan, will end up with you not feeling very good and your health suffering.

Below, we are going to spend some time talking about the nutrients that you need to consider if you plan to go on a plant-based diet. In fact, these nutrients can be important even if you are not on the vegan diet or other plant-based diets. It is possible that even as an omnivore, you can be deficient of these nutrients, so avoiding animal products is not necessarily the problem here.

The problem that comes up here is that we are not eating enough of the healthy and whole plant-based foods. This is where the plant-based diet comes into play. It helps you to eat a wider range of whole plant-based foods, along with some healthy carbs, to help you fill in those micronutrients that you have been missing out on.

While there are a lot of different micronutrients that you need to make sure to add to the body, there are four major ones that are considered the most important for vegans to consider getting. These include B12, vitamin D, omega-3 DHA, EPA, and iodine. You also want to make sure that you get nutrients like vitamin A, vitamin K, magnesium, zinc, iron, and calcium as well.

Vitamin B12

The first nutrient we are going to take a look at is Vitamin B12. This is synthesized by bacteria that is found in dirt and soil. It is a common misconception that it only comes from animal secretions like milk and eggs and animal flesh. But it is possible to get these from other sources as well. You need to make sure that you are getting enough of this nutrient though since it is so important for the synthesis of DNA, for neurological function, and for red blood formation.

Since the soil is often depleted of this nutrient, and we often wash our fruits and vegetables anyway, it is hard to get enough of the B12 vitamin into our day. Because of this, it is often recommended that you supplement this vitamin into your diet when you are a vegan. This is the only vitamin that is not going to be readily available in your foods, but you can sometimes find in foods that have been fortified, like cereals.

Omega-3 DHA and EPA

Note that the RDA for overall omega-3 fatty acids and there isn't a recommended daily amount for the EPA and DHA on their own. But with that said, the American Heart Foundation recommends that you consume about 500 mg of these combined per day, and then there are studies that recommend a bit more, saying that 1000 mg per day of DHA and 220 mg per day of EPA is the best.

These fatty acids are important for the absorption of nutrients in the body, for the health of your brain, and for an overall level of optimal health. They also have a nice healing effect on the body and have properties that can prevent inflammation. If there is a lack of omega-3 in the diet, it can cause issues like mood imbalances, digestive health, auto-immune disease, depression, and brain damage.

Since most people know that they should get these omega-3 fatty acids from fish, how is the vegan supposed to maintain their diet plan and still see the results? Some of the best foods that you can consume that are vegan friendly and high in both the DHA and EPA of omega-3 fatty acids include:

1. Wild rice
2. Mangos and berries
3. Leafy greens
4. Vegetables like sprouts, broccoli, and cauliflower
5. Winter squash
6. Legumes
7. Chia seeds
8. Seeds and nuts
9. Seaweed
10. Hemp seed
11. Walnuts
12. Flaxseed

Vitamin K2

This is an important vitamin because it helps with the functioning of your kidneys, your brain health, your bone health, and with blood clotting. This one is pretty easy to find when you are on the vegan diet, as long as you take in enough fruits and vegetables along the way.

When we are looking at vitamin K, we will find that it comes in two varieties. Vitamin K1, the primary and most natural form of vitamin K that we obtain through plants, and vitamin K2, the one that is produced by intestinal bacteria. K2 is really important because it is helpful to the health of your bones and can help to move calcium around the body.

There are a lot of foods you can consume in order to get the amounts of vitamin K2 that your body needs when you are on the vegan diet and these include:

1. Swiss chard

2. Wheat Bran
3. Kiwi
4. Leafy greens, especially spinach
5. Pumpkin
6. Okra
7. Edamame
8. Broccoli
9. Turnips
10. Kale and cabbage
11. Fermented soy products

Vitamin A

The next vitamin that you need to focus on when you are on this kind of diet plan is vitamin A. Even though there are a lot of great sources of this vitamin when you are on this diet plan, it is still important to focus on it a bit. Studies have shown that it takes as much as 12 micrograms of beta-carotene to produce one microgram of vitamin A. This makes it super important to really load up on foods that are full of beta-carotene to take care of your vitamin A.

The good news is that this is possible. You should also try to combine these foods that are rich in vitamin A with fats in order to improve the absorption. Adding a bit of avocado, seeds, and nuts to your meals can be a great way to do this.

Some of the foods that are amazing when it comes to providing your body with the vitamin A that it needs include:

1. Collard Greens
2. Apricots
3. Carrots
4. Spinach
5. Kale
6. Cantaloupe
7. Butternut squash
8. Sweet potato

Vitamin D

This is an important nutrient to work on because it is going to play a role in the absorption of calcium and in cell growth. Being deficient in this can be linked back to weak bones, depression, muscle weakness, and cancer. This vitamin can cause a deficiency in anyone on any meal plan because most people are not absorbing it through the sun as they should.

There are not as many foods on the vegan diet that naturally come with vitamin D in them. And if you live somewhere that is cold for a good portion of the year, it can be hard to get this nutrient from the sun. During the summer months, though, just spending half an hour outside in the sun can help you get the vitamin D that you need.

If you aren't planning on supplementing this vitamin D, then you need to look for plant versions of this to help you out. Some of the options you can go with include:

1. All the different kinds of mushrooms.
2. Fortified tofu and any soy products that are fermented.
3. Fortified cereals.
4. Almond and soy milks that are fortified.

Iodine

This is more of a trace element that the body needs in order to produce the hormones of the thyroid. This can be very important to bone and brain development and to your metabolism. Being deficient in this trace element can cause insufficient hormone production from the thyroid, which can lead to a whole host of issues. There are some smaller studies that show how vegans could be at a greater risk for lower iodine intake than others, but it is something that is easy for you to take care of once you know the problem.

Salt is a good way to add in some more iodine to your diet. You will probably be fine with your iodine intake if you add just a bit of salt to your meals on a regular basis. Adding in some seaweed to your diet can provide you with more of the iodine that you need as well.

Calcium

This is another option that is not too hard to get when you are on the vegan diet, but it is still something that you need to be aware of and you need to ensure that you are consuming plenty of these foods each day. And if you are able to consume it along with vitamin D, that is even better.

Calcium is important for your heart function and your muscle functions, for enzyme reactions, nerve impulses, and blood flow. There are a number of different foods that you can consume that will help you to get the calcium that you need including:

1. Beans
2. Broccoli
3. Almonds
4. Tempeh
5. Quinoa
6. Kale
7. Dried figs
8. Fortified plant juices and milk
9. Almonds and almond butter

Other important nutrients

We have spent some time talking about all of the great nutrients that you should consider adding into your diet, and the different foods that you are going to be able to eat to get these nutrients. As long as you eat a varied diet that is high in many nutrients, you are going to see results with the vegan diet and feel amazing. But some of the other types of nutrients and minerals that you need to ensure find their way into this diet plan include:

1. Zinc
2. Magnesium
3. Iron
4. Sulfur
5. Creatine
6. Beta-alanine
7. Carnonsine

Eating a diet that is full of good plants and produce, and some great whole wheats and more will help you get all of these great nutrients and more into your diet plan. If you get stuck eating the same foods from one day to the next, this is where you will start losing out on some of the healthy nutrients, including the ones above, that your body needs so much of. But when you mix things up and add in some variety, you will find that it is so much easier to work with this diet plan and stay healthy and feel amazing.

Chapter 3: Are There Any Deficiencies to Worry About?

One major problem that many people worry about when they are on a vegan diet is whether they are going to run into any deficiencies. They worry that they are not going to be able to get the vitamins and nutrients that their body needs since they are cutting down some major food groups and aren't eating them any longer.

For the most part, as long as you are making sure that you eat a varied diet with lots of plant-based foods that are good and healthy for you, you are going to do just fine with being on this kind of diet plan. However, there are times when you may need to supplement on this a little bit, especially if you are new to the diet plan and haven't worked with this kind of eating plan in the past.

Vegan and vegetarian diets alike can be really beneficial to your overall health. But you have to remember that completely going through and cutting out animal products could make you question whether you are getting the nutrients that you need.

It is common to assume that you are going to be low on protein when you go on this kind of diet, but this is often not the nutrient that you need to worry about. There are lots of different protein sources that you can consume when you are a vegan, without having to eat animal products. These include options like whole grains, soy products, nuts and seeds, chickpeas, beans, and lentils.

There are a few nutrients that are easy to miss out on when you decide to follow this kind of diet plan though. Knowing what these are and why they are so important can make a big difference in your overall health. Some of the most common deficiencies that come up on the vegetarian and vegan diet include:

1. Vitamin B12: This is a vitamin that is very important and is easily found in many of the animal products that you ate before. But, the good news is that there are many plant-based foods that have been fortified with this nutrient, such as cereals, plant milks, and nutritional yeast, so you should be fine. If you are worried about getting this one, adding a supplement can help.
2. Vitamin D: This is also known as the sunshine vitamin. Along with calcium, it plays a big role in keeping your bones healthy. This nutrient is easy to get if you are able to get yourself out in the sun. Supplementation can be helpful for those who live up north and can't get out as much.

3. The omega-3 fatty acids: This is a very important fatty acid that can help keep your heart as healthy as possible. While eggs and fish are often thought to be rich sources of omega-3 fatty acids, you are able to get these through hempseeds, walnuts, flaxseeds, and chia seeds.
4. Zinc: This can be found in whole grains, legumes, and many beans. It is important to note that the phytic acids that are sometimes found in plants can hinder the absorption of zinc. If you soak or sprout beans and grains before you cook, you can work on solving this problem.
5. Iron: Even though the iron that comes from plants won't be absorbed as easily as other sources, eating a diet that is varied and has lots of plant-based foods should be enough to ensure that you get iron. You will be able to find this iron in

places like dried fruits, peas, lentils, whole grains, and leafy green vegetables. Adding foods rich in vitamin C to this can help you absorb the iron a lot easier.

Eating a varied and healthy diet is the best way to ensure that you are able to keep your body healthy, and to ensure that you are not dealing with a nutrient deficiency. It is sometimes hard to work with a plant-based diet and also worry about your nutrition. But if you are looking to go on this diet plan to lose weight or to improve your overall health, then these are the things that you need to focus on. Many beginners find that working with supplementation in the beginning as they adjust helps. But you can certainly get through this diet plan and stay healthy, while getting the nutrients that you need, without the supplementation.

Chapter 4: Everything You Need to Know About Meal Planning

When it comes to meal planning, you are going to quickly notice that it can make a big difference when it is time to stick to a dietary change in your life. While it is easy to head out to a restaurant or make a freezer meal that is unhealthy when your family is hungry, it fills you up with a lot of junk that is not good for the body and can make your wallet shrink way too fast.

Meal planning can solve the issue of being too busy or not knowing how you will have time to make a meal when you have a million things going on during the day. Just pick one day a week to get everything done, and then your meals are ready whenever you are for the week, or a few weeks, or however long you would like. It helps you to save time and money and ensures that your family is able to eat healthy, no matter which diet plan you are on.

The benefits of meal planning

Meal planning is going to be one of the most important aspects of eating a diet that is healthy, and there are actually quite a few benefits to doing this. Even if you have been eating healthy for a long time, this process can really make life easier and will ensure you stay with your dietary goals for the whole week. There are so many benefits that come with meal planning, and some of the biggest ones include:

It saves money. There are always going to be times when money is tight, or when we just want to save some money on our grocery bill. Meal planning can help out with this. First, you will not spend so much time and money eating out. Since it can easily cost $30 or more to take your family out for one meal you can imagine the savings you can make when you prepare whole meals that are healthy for your family for $10 or less!

There will also be less food waste in the long run. When you aren't grabbing groceries with no plans for them, and letting them sit there and go bad, you won't have as much waste, which can save money. Meal planning allows you to know exactly how much of each item of food you need, and you can work from there to save more money as well. Add on some bulk shopping and picking meals that share some items can make things even easier.

You get the benefit of eating real food on a meal plan. When you consume a diet that is rich in nutrients, like you find on the vegan diet, it is going to be so good for all aspects of your health. But you do need to plan some things ahead of time. Meal planning can help with this because it lets you decide before you go into the store what meals you will eat during the week. You can purchase healthy ingredients, and know that you will actually use them!

Those who decide to meal plan end up wasting less food overall. How many times have you gone out with the best intentions of eating something, and a month or so later, you find bags of fruits and vegetables that were shoved to the back of the fridge and forgotten because you didn't know what to do with them? This is a waste of time and money and can be so frustrating. Making a meal plan, and purchasing the items that you need for that, can ensure that there is less waste.

Many people enjoy meal planning because it leads to less stress. It is really stressful when at four in the evening, you realize that it is almost supper time and you have nothing planned for dinner. And the general worry about what to cook for supper will be at the back of your head all the time. Making a meal plan and sticking to it can make a big difference in how great you feel, and how much less stress you have at the last minute each night.

Even though you do need to sit down and come up with a meal plan each week, it can save you time. Planning ahead allows you to cook things in bulk and then you can save some for later for a different meal. And you can pre-plan out your meals to do the instant pot or slow cooker to save even more time.

And finally, you are going to enjoy that this meal plan makes it easy to add some variety to your diet plan. Many people worry that meal planning is going to be boring and rigid. But according to statistics, families who don't meal plan are the ones who end up eating the same meals over and over again. Meal planning makes it easier to mix things up since you can look it up and think it through ahead of time.

Tips to make meal planning easier

Meal planning doesn't have to be hard, as long as you have a nice system in place for it. But there are a few things that you need to keep in mind so that you are able to get started on this process and see the best results in no time. Some of these include:

Have a daily template that you can use. Rather than having to start from nothing each week, you can work on a template of the general types of foods that you are going to cook each day of the week and the number of times that you will use each main food. You may have a fish meal, a slow cooker meal, a salad, and a few stir fry's for example. This guidebook has six weeks of meals all planned out for you to make life easier, but you can sort things out, once the meal plan is done, to make this easier.

Next, you can focus on core recipes. Once you are able to find some core recipes that your family seems to enjoy, save them, and reuse them every few weeks. If you are able to find 20 of these or so, that is enough to get through most of the month, and you won't be as bored with your meals any longer. Each week, use these core meals for five of the dinners and then add in something new for a few. If you are really motivated for this, you can build up 20 core meals that go with each season, and then use seasonal produce that goes with them to save more money.

Stretching out your protein can work as well. Protein is often going to be the most expensive part of any meal so try to work with cuts that are not as expensive, and then stretch it out. This can help you out a lot. The cuts of meat in the vegan diet are not going to be as important, but finding ways to cut costs on tofu and other protein sources that you do use can make a world of difference as well.

Always remember to mix in some spices if you can. This works on pretty much any diet plan as long as you make sure that you aren't adding in a lot of preservatives and salt to them. You can change up the taste of a recipe by changing the spices that you are using. If you are running out of ideas on what you would like to cook, consider just mixing up the spices a bit and you will notice a big difference.

Traveling the world can be a lot of fun when making meals. Even if you can't afford to go all over the world, you can certainly mix it up in your home and have different meals throughout the week, and your meal plan will make this so much easier. Maybe have Mexican one night, Chinese on another, and so on. You may find that your children actually like the mix-up and it opens the world to a lot of new recipes that you are able to try out and see what they do for you.

Never become a short order cook though. While meal planning frees up your time, it is fine to ask family members to give their input on what they would like to eat. This isn't an excuse for you to make ten different meals throughout the day. Pick out different meals and take the tastes of your family into consideration. But if they all want something different, that is just too bad. Quitting this habit can save you money, make meal planning easier, and help to avoid issues with picky eaters in your family as they grow up.

And finally, when you are planning out this meal plan, remember to think about the leftovers a bit. You can save yourself some cooking time, and reduce waste when you decide to eat more leftovers in your day. It can be tough to break out of the mindset that you need to make a new meal all the time, but it isn't necessary. Save yourself the headache, and make grocery shopping easier when you eat some leftovers on a regular basis.

Following a meal plan is one of the best things that you can do for your home. It allows you to release some of the stress, can make it easier to follow a good diet plan (even a vegan one) and helps you to save money in the long run. Sure, it takes a bit of your time at the beginning of the week (or you can do this every few weeks to really get ahead of the game), but it can be so worth it.

Steps to meal planning

Before we move on to some of the foods you can consider for a vegan diet, and some of the best recipes, it is important to know the basic steps that come with meal planning and how you can get started. Meal planning is a very simple process that you can use to improve your overall health and well-being, but it is going to take some time and patience to make it happen. Some of the steps that you can follow to get started with meal planning include:

1. Pick out your meals: You need to sit down and plan out the meals that you want to use for the week. Make sure to plan out breakfasts, lunches, dinners, and snacks so that you aren't scrambling around. You can look online for ideas, or look through cookbooks and other resources. Consider looking at specific resources for the vegan diet when you want to follow this one.

2. Make a grocery list. Once you have picked out and written down the recipes that you would like to work with, it is time to move on and focus on writing a grocery list. Write down everything that you are going to need for the week. This can save you trips back and forth to the

grocery store. Just remember to take your list with you!

3. Shop only for what you need. Getting sidetracked at the store is going to cause you to make poor decisions, forget things, and can make staying on this kind of diet more difficult.

4. Prep as much as you can ahead of time. You may want to do this on a second day so as not to overwhelm yourself. But taking some time to prep as much of the food ahead of time can make life easier. Slice up the vegetables, and prepare as much as you can. If you are able to put together most of the meal and freeze it, that is even better.

5. Enjoy. When the time comes to eat the meal, most of the work should be done. You may have to throw a few things together or put something in the oven, but you will be glad to see that most of

the work, if you did it properly, was done ahead of time.

And that is all there is to it! Meal planning takes some organization in order to see the results, but you will find that it is going to be one of the best choices that you can make when going on the vegan diet or any diet plan for that matter. It is easy to follow, fun to work with, and can open up so many new recipes that you are bound to enjoy as well!

Chapter 5:Nutrient Dense Vegan Foods to Get Started

As a vegan, you are cutting out a few major food groups that can provide you with the nutrients that you need. This means that every bite is really going to count when you go on this diet plan. It is perfectly possible to get all the nutrients that your body needs when you go vegan, but you can't waste your calories with baked goods and other things that don't pack that nutrition in.

The good news is that there are a lot of great tasting foods that you can add to your vegan diet that will pack a nutritional punch, and ensure that you aren't going to fall into a nutrient deficiency in the process. Some of the best foods to add to your diet to improve your health will include:

1. Kale: Kale is one of the best foods that you can consume when you are on a vegan diet. It is going to contain 200 percent of your vitamin C, 300 percent of your Vitamin A and 1000 percent of your Vitamin K. It also includes other nutrients that you need including manganese, copper, magnesium, calcium, potassium, fiber, and vitamin B6.
2. Watercress: This one is similar to kale, and it can actually help reduce the DNA damage that may occur in blood cells thanks to free radicals. It also includes the nutrients that you need to maintain connective tissue that is good, protects against infections, can reduce the damage to neurons, and strengthen the bones.
3. Bok Choy: This one is has lots of vitamin B6, which is important for metabolizing fat, protein, and carbs, and it can also

provide you with potassium that helps with nerve function and your muscle functions as well.

4. Spinach: This is a good leafy green that is high in so many things that it should be added to your diet on most days. In this one, you will find things like manganese, copper, phosphorus, magnesium, iron, calcium, folate, vitamin B6, thiamin, Vitamins A, C, E, and K, fiber, and protein!

5. Brussels Sprouts:This vegetable contains some of the cholesterol-lowering benefits that you need and is also high in fiber. Brussels Sprouts can also help to improve the stability of DNA in white blood cells when you consume them on a regular basis.

6. Strawberries: They have a ton of antioxidants that can protect your heart against any disease, regulate your blood sugar levels, and even fight against

cancer and reduce your risk of developing type 2 diabetes.

7. Flaxseeds: These are a great option to go for when looking to get the omega-3 fatty acids that we were talking about earlier. They also contain something known as lignans, which are compounds that are like fiber and can provide you some protection. These seeds help with arthritis, inflammatory bowel disease, and heart disease.

8. Cherries: This is another good fruit to go with on this diet plan. They are full of antioxidants and can help to repair and even prevent some of the damage that can happen to the body thanks to free radicals. There are a ton of benefits to eating cherries, including protecting against cancers, fighting inflammation, and protecting the heart. Plus they taste really good.

These are just a few of the different types of foods that you are able to enjoy when you go on the vegan diet. Make sure that you pick out a wide variety of foods, and add a bunch of color to your plate, rather than just eating the same foods from one day to the next. This will ensure that you provide your body with the nutrients that it needs, even when you are following this kind of diet plan.

Chapter 6: How to Store Your Food

One thing that you need to consider when it is time to work on vegan meal planning is how you are going to store all of your food. You may take a look at the meal plan and the recipes that we have in this guidebook, and be ready to start. But once you have all of that food, what are you going to do with it?

Meal planning is not just about picking up some of the ingredients and calling it good. It also focuses on helping you prep and get things ready ahead of time so that you are able to just throw a few things together and have meals ready. But once you do all of this, you need to make sure that you store the food properly so that it lasts, and remains good and fresh when you are ready to eat it.

This chapter is going to take some time to look at the different things that you can consider when it comes to storing your food while meal planning. We will look at how to freeze your food, the importance of avoiding containers that have BPA in them to protect your health, and more!

Freezing the meals

One of the best things that you can do to prepare with meal planning is to freeze your meals. This can be great if you would like to plan out more than one week at a time. You can make some of the meals that you need, and freeze them until you need them. Think about how easy it will be when you are in a rush one night, and you can just reach into your freezer and pull out a delicious meal that just needs to be heated up!

Changing up the meals and making them work for freezer meals can be super easy. Many of the meals that you make can be turned into freezer meals. If it is a casserole, you just need to make it and put it into the freezer when it cools down. If it is something that has to be mixed together, prepare the vegetables and everything else, and then just pull out all those ingredients when you are ready to make it.

The more that you are able to prepare ahead of time, the easier meal planning is going to be for you. And if you are able to freeze some of the ingredients, it will make your life that much easier as well. You can store them there for longer, allowing you to meal plan more than one week at a time, and can just make life easier and healthier overall.

Pantry items

When it comes to pantry items, you probably don't need to worry about these too much. If you haven't opened them up yet, then there are no worries about them going bad too quickly. You should do a periodic check of your pantry though to make sure that the foods in there are still good and that you aren't eating things that are out of date and bad for you.

If you do happen to open up something in the pantry, make sure that you are able to seal it up when you are done or put it in another container or bag to help keep it sealed. Leaving any food open can make it go bad over time, and it invites ants and other creatures into your home. Keep the food safe and sealed so that you can use it and not waste it.

Why is BPA bad for you?

There are a lot of different products out there that are meant to help you store some of the foods that you are making with meal planning, and ensure that you can keep them in the fridge or the freezer until you need them. But one thing that you need to be aware of is that many of these products contain BPA, which is something you definitely need to avoid.

BPA is a chemical that has been added to a lot of commercial products, including the hygiene products and the containers that you use on a regular basis. This chemical was discovered in the 1890s, and was then used along with other compounds in the 1950s to make strong and resilient plastics. These plastics are now used for many items including baby bottles and food containers.

There are a lot of different products in our modern world that contain this BPA and they include:

1. Dental filling sealants

2. A lot of the sports equipment that we use
3. Eyeglass lenses
4. Household electronics
5. Thermal printer receipts
6. Feminine hygiene products
7. Toiletries
8. Canned foods
9. Any items that have been put in plastic containers.

It is also important to note that many of the products that say are free from BPA have just been replaced with either bisphenol-S or bisphenol-F. However, even small concentrations of these chemicals are going to be bad for you and could cause some disruptions to your cells like the BPA is. It is important to avoid containers and other products that have these chemicals to keep your body safe and functioning in the proper way.

Now, you may ask how BPA enters your body. The main source of exposure to this chemical is through your diet. When containers with BPA are made, not all of the BPA is sealed inside that product. This means that some of it can break free and mix with the contents of the container they are added into.

For instance, a recent study found that the levels of BPA in urine decreased by 66 percent following three days during which the participants stopped eating packaged foods. Then in another study, there were people who ate either a canned or fresh soup each day for five days. The urine levels of BPA for these participants were more than 1221 percent high.

The next thing to discuss is whether BPA is really that bad for you. To look at this, we need to take some time to look at how BPA works and why it may be harmful and something that you need to be careful of.

It is believed that BPA is able to mimic the function and the structure of the estrogen hormone. Because it is similar to estrogen in shape, it is possible for the BPA to bind to the estrogen receptors and can influence a lot of the processes in the body including reproduction, energy levels, fetal development, cell repair, and growth. In addition, this chemical is able to interact with some of the other hormone receptors, such as those of the thyroid, and can alter those functions.

You will find that your body is extremely sensitive to changes in hormone levels. When BPA is able to mimic estrogen and cause some damage, it can cause some negative effects to your health. And, the more BPA that ends up in your body, the worse the problem with your hormones is going to get.

With the information above in mind, you may find that a lot of people think that the use of BPA should be banned. There are several places where BPA is restricted, including Malaysia, China, Canada, and the EU. Some states in the United States have followed this, but as of yet, there are no federal regulations in place.

In the year 2014, the FDA released its latest report, which helped to confirm the original 1980s daily exposure limit of 23 mcg per pound of body weight, and concluded that BPA is probably safe at the levels that companies are allowed to use, right now. However, there is mounting research that shows that even these levels may be too high and that some changes need to be made. In one recent study, rodents were able to show the negative effects of BPA at levels as low as 4.5 mcg per pound each day.

What's more, research that has been done in monkeys shows that levels equivalent to those currently measured in humans have a negative effect on the reproduction of the person consuming it. It is believed that BPA is able to affect several different aspects of your fertility, which can be bad for those who want to get pregnant or who would like to do so in the future.

One study observed that women who had frequent miscarriages had three times as much BPA found in their blood compared to women who had successful pregnancies. In addition, studies on women who were going through fertility treatments showed that those who had BPA at higher levels had proportionally lower egg production, and were actually, because of these BPA levels, two times less likely to become pregnant.

Among couples who were going through IVF treatments, those who had the highest levels of BPA in the group were at least 30 percent more likely to produce embryos that would be classified as lower quality. In another study, it was found that men who had high levels of BPA ended up being up to 4 times more likely to have a low sperm count and concentration.

This goes even further. One study took a look at men who worked at a local BPA manufacturing company in China. Of these, it was more than 4 times more likely that they suffered from less satisfaction with sex and erectile difficulty compared to other men who were similar except for their workspace.

While these are really notable effects, there are several recent reviews that agree that before we jump on the bandwagon with this, we need to take a look at the evidence a bit more and see if we are able to find out more about BPA and confirm the results ahead of time.

With that said, there are several health risks that come with consuming too much BPA in your diet. These can include:

1. Higher risk of heart disease
2. Type 2 diabetes
3. Raises your risk of obesity
4. PCOS: BPA ended up being up to 46 percent higher in women with this condition compared to others.
5. Premature delivery: Women who took in more BPA during their pregnancy were up to 92 percent more likely to have their baby before 37 weeks.
6. Asthma: Higher exposure to BPA can increase the risk of up to 130 percent of wheezing in infants who are younger than six months old.
7. Liver functions: These higher levels show that there is a 29 percent higher risk of abnormal liver enzyme levels.

8. Issues with the immune function: BPA levels are going to contribute to the immune system not working as well.
9. Thyroid function: Higher BPA levels are going to be linked back to issues with thyroid hormones and can show that the thyroid isn't working that well.
10. Brain functionWith studies showing how bad BPA is for us, you may wish to avoid products that have BPA when you are doing your meal planning. There are a few ways that you can do this and ensure that your exposure is kept to a minimum as much as possible. Some of these include:
1. Avoid food that is packaged: This is something that is easy to do when you are on the vegan diet. Avoid foods that are packaged in plastic containers, anything with recycling numbers of 7 and 3, and any canned foods.

2. Drink from a glass bottle: You should buy liquids in a glass bottle rather than cans and plastic bottles.
3. Stay away from any products with BPA: As much as you can, try to limit your contact with things like receipts because they contain BPA as well.
4. Don't microwave your plastic containers: If you are going to microwave your food, do it in glass rather than plastic.

When it comes to meal planning, it is best if you are able to find containers that are free of BPA and that will help you to get this done and keep things safe. If you can find glass containers or other containers that do not contain BPA, use them so that you can get all the health benefits of the vegan diet and from meal planning, without all of the bad stuff.

Chapter 7: Staples In Every Vegans Kitchen

Congratulations on becoming a vegan! This is an exciting time to improve your health and work to see the best benefits possible. When it comes to meal planning on this diet plan, there are a lot of different items that you are going to need to add to your pantry, many of which you may have never had before. This is a very different meal plan compared to the one that you were following before. And having a few of the staples around ahead of time, and filling up your pantry, can make a big difference in how easy it is to stay on this kind of meal plan. Some of the staples that are found in every vegans kitchen include:

1. Legumes: Whether you decide to go with ones that are canned or dry, you should always make sure that you have

a variety of beans in your pantry. You can also consider going with some options.

2. Rolled Oatmeal. Oatmeal is a good breakfast to have when you are on the vegetarian diet, and you will find that a lot of the breakfasts that are available in our meal plans will include this staple as well. You can even add them to cookies and more! Keep a few rolled oats on hand.

3. Whole grains: You will be able to enjoy a lot of whole grains when it comes to following this diet plan. You will want to make sure that you have a wide variety of these on hand as well. The best ones to have on standby include couscous, farro, millet, quinoa, and rice. You can keep a few of these and other options around to make life easier.

4. Flours: Whether you love to bake some fun treats while on this diet plan or not,

you will find that having some flour options on hand can help. If you want to go gluten-free, make sure to keep some of that on hand as well, but it isn't necessary while being vegan.

5. Seeds: Seeds are popular on this diet plan as well and it is a good idea to keep several varieties on hand in case you want to add them to something. You may want to choose a few options like sesame seeds, sunflower seeds, chia seeds, hemp seeds, and flax seeds.

6. Nuts: While you are on a vegan diet, you will most likely consume some type of nut each day. You can even enjoy them in the form of some nut butters to add some healthy protein and fat, and a bit of flavor and texture to your meals. And they work great for an extra snack if you need it.

7. Nutritional yeast: You will find that many of the recipes that we use in this

guidebook are going to include nutritional yeast. You are going to use this for so many things, that it is important to make sure that you keep some on hand.

8. Salt: Don't forget to keep some salt on hand. This is a great way to season up some of the meals that you are making. And since it keeps well, you won't have to worry about it fading and not being good in a short amount of time.

9. Coconut oil: This is one of the best oils, along with olive oil, to keep around in your kitchen thanks to all of the nutrients that are found in it. You can use it for baking, frying, and so much more and you will love the nice flavor that comes with it.

10. Olive oil:Don't forget about all of the healthy things that you can get out of olive oil and the great nutrition that is found inside. This and coconut oil

should always be found in your pantry when you are a vegan. Try to get the highest quality olive oil that you can though because it contains more of the healthy fats that you need to help you out.

11. Maple syrup: This is one of the best sweeteners that you can use when you decide to go on this kind of diet. It is going to be great with any kind of baked goods, as a topping on any waffles or pancakes that you make, and even on granola.
12. Sriracha: This is a great hot sauce that works well on many meals, and you will find it in this guidebook quite a bit. And it often doesn't upset stomachs like other hot sauces can, making it one of the best options for you to choose.
13. Onions and garlic: These two are going to be found in a lot of the foods that you choose to go with, and they have a ton of

flavor, without all of the expense. You will be able to add them to get more flavor and texture to your meals, so keep some on hand.

14. Lemons: This is another way to brighten up almost any of the dishes that you will enjoy on this diet plan, and it is also beneficial to your whole body. You will find that adding a bit of lemon juice to your water can help to increase your energy, fight off bloating, balance your appetite, and give you clearer skin than ever before.

15. Avocados: If you are looking for a great item that can go into many meals, and give you the healthy fats that you desire, and tastes good, then this is the food that you need to add to your pantry. Whether you eat them regularly, mash them up, or make guacamole with them, avocados can be a great addition to your meals!

16. Mushrooms: There are so many great recipes out there that utilize mushrooms, and it is a shame not to just keep some on hand! There is so much taste, texture, and versatility that comes with having some on hand, and it can make a difference in how easy it is to get your meal planning done.
17. Baby carrots: Whether you need an easy snack to enjoy on the vegan diet or you need to add something to one of your main dishes, baby carrots are the perfect addition. Add in some hummus and you are going to have a great snack to enjoy as well. You can choose to eat these raw or steam and cook them up to make them nice and soft.
18. Greens: As you go through some of the recipes that we talk about in this guidebook, you will find that there is an abundance of greens that are encouraged. All types of greens from

lettuce to spinach to kale and more can work well on this diet plan, filling you up between meals and making it easier to get all of the healthy nutrition that your body needs. Try to keep a few different kinds on hand when you are making your meals.

19. Almond milk: This is often the favorite when it comes to non-dairy milks that work on the vegan diet. It is able to go with pretty much anything that you need to make including baked goods, pancakes and waffles, smoothies, oatmeal, and cereal. You can even drink it plain if you need to get some extra calcium in your day.

20. Tofu: You will find that when it comes to the vegan diet, tofu is going to be super important to work with. This is a very versatile food that can be baked, fried, and scrambled and can give you a filling and tasty meal. You can even use

it in place of some eggs in many of your baked goods to give you an even better product. This also works as the main part of the meal, for sour cream, dressings, creamy sauces, and even tofu cheese if you wish.

21. Spices: When it comes to being a vegan, spices are going to become your new best friend. Make sure to add in as many of the different spices as you can. The grocery lists that we will provide in this guidebook will have lots of spices to add to your meals, so when you follow that, you will naturally be able to fill up your pantry with a ton of delicious and easy to use spices. Go with as much variety as you can. A simple change in the spice that you decide to use can change up a whole dish. Some good options are cinnamon, turmeric, chili pepper, garlic powder, and more.

22. Potatoes and sweet potatoes: These are both good things to add to a meal when you want some flavor and filling. Both are versatile enough to work with almost any other ingredient that you would like to combine. Put these in soups or have them as the main dish, and you will be amazed at the results that you are able to get in the process.

As you can see, there are a lot of different foods that you can consider when it comes to working on a vegan meal plan. Filling up your pantry can take some time, and you may find that as you try out some recipes and experiment a bit, you will need to add a few other staples to your main pantry to keep you ready for anything. But adding in a few of these ingredients and keeping them well stocked will do wonders when it comes to helping you get started with meal planning, even when you are on the vegan diet.

Chapter 8: Week One Meal Plan and Grocery List

The Meal Plan

Day 1	Day 2:	Day 3:	Day 4:
Breakfast: Pumpkin Steel Cut Oats Lunch: Green Pea Risotto Dinner: Chickpea Salad Snack: Risotto Bites	Breakfast: Cinnamon Overnight Oats Lunch: Yummy Potatoes and Kale Dinner: Warm Quinoa Salad Snack: Kale Chips	Breakfast: Breakfast Bowls Lunch: Warm Vegetable Salad Dinner: Black Bean Soup Snack: Taco Pita Pizzas	Breakfast: Sweet Potato Hash Lunch: Not Tuna Salad Dinner: Pineapple Quinoa Salad Snack: Seed Crackers
Day 5	Day 6:	Day 7:	

Breakfast: Green Smoothie Lunch: Red Bean and Corn Salad Dinner: Butternut Squash Gnocchi Snack: Tamari Almonds	Breakfast: Tortilla Breakfast Casserole Lunch: Mediterranean Beans and Greens Dinner: BBQ Sandwich Snack: Roasted Chickpeas	Breakfast: Smoothie Breakfast Bowl Lunch: Cheesy Polenta Dinner: NO Cook Quesadilla Snack: Veggie Pinwheels	

The Grocery List

½ c. Panko Bread crumbs	2 buns	4 Pita Beads
10 corn tortillas	5 tortillas	1 tbsp. Agave Nectar
1 ¾ c. cornmeal	¼ c. chia seeds	½ c. Sesame Seeds
2 ½ c. maple syrup	¾ c. nutritional yeast	1 c. baked granola
2 ½ cups rolled oats	1 c. Steel Cut Oats	2 cans black beans
2 cans cannellini beans	2 cans and 3 c. chickpeas	1 can great northern beans
2 cans Kidney beans	1 c. refried beans	¼ c. green olives
¾ cup hummus	1 c. Pizza sauce	9 c. vegetable broth
1/3 cup tahini	½ cup vegan cheddar	1 c. vegan queso

½ c. vegan mayo	12 tbsp. Olive oil	Cooking spray
1 cup salsa	½ c. Vegan BBQ	2 tsp. vegan Worcestershire
4 tbsp. Tamari Sauce	3 tsp. vegan butter	1 ¼ c. cashew cream
18 c. plant based milk	¼ c. basil	1 tsp. cayenne pepper
3 tsp. chili powder	2 tsp. chipotle powder	1/3 c. cilantro
1 tsp. ground cinnamon	2 tsp. cumin	2 tsp. dill
1 tsp. garlic powder	1 tsp. oregano	1 tsp. paprika
½ c. parsley	Salt	Pepper
1 tsp. ground turmeric	1 can hearts of palm	1 c. couscous
4 c. gnocchi	2.5 c. barley	5 c. quinoa
1 c. Arborio rice	10 oz. Arugula	1 avocado
8 bananas	2 c. berries	2 lbs. carrots
½ c. celery	3 Swiss chard	1 ½ cherries

	leaves	
2 c. corn	1 cucumber	1 c. dragon fruit
9 tsp. minced garlic	4 garlic cloves	4 c. mixed greens
6 oz. kale	1 lemon	6 Tbsp. and ½ cc. lemon juice
Romain lettuce (8 c.)	3 limes	3 c. mushrooms
¼ red onion	½ white onion	2 c. peas
Jalapeno	1. pineapple	1 c. pomegranate seeds
2 Russet potatoes	4 red potatoes	½ c. pumpkin puree
4 c. spinach	2 c. tofu	½ butternut squash
4 c. hulled strawberries	1 can diced tomatoes	1 block tofu
1 lb. raw almonds	5 tbsp. Chopped pecans	1 c. pumpkin seeds
Sunflower seeds ½ c.		

The Recipes

Breakfast

Pumpkin Steel Cut Oats

Servings: 4

What's inside:

Salt
Maple syrup (2 tbsp.)
Pumpkin seeds (.25 c.)
Pumpkin puree (.5 c.)
Steel-cut oats (1 c.)
Water (3 c.)

How to make:

1. Bring some water to boil in a pan. When the water is hot, add in the oats and stir. Reduce the heat to a low setting.
2. After 30 minutes of simmering, the oats will be soft. Add in the pumpkin puree.
3. Cook for another five minutes and then add in the maple syrup, pumpkin seeds, and salt.
4. Divide into four bowls and serve.

Cinnamon Overnight Oats

What's inside:

Ground ginger (1 tsp.)
Ground cinnamon (1 tsp.)
Salt (1 tsp.)
Maple syrup (2.5 tsp.)
Unsweetened plant based milk (5 c.)
Chopped pecans (5 Tbsp.)
Pumpkin seeds (5 Tbsp.)
Rolled oats (2.5 c.)

How to make

1. Bring out five pint jars. In each one, add in a pinch of ginger, pinch of cinnamon, pinch of salt, half a teaspoon of maple syrup, a cup of milk, one tablespoon of pecans and pumpkin seeds, and half a cup of oats.
2. Stir these ingredients. Close with some lids and serve with fresh fruit if you wish.

Breakfast Bowls

What's inside:

Slivered almonds (2 tbsp.)
Vanilla plant based milk (3 c.)
Cherries, dried (1.5 c.)
Salt
Water (3.25 c.)
Pearl barley (1.5 c.)

How to make:

1. Take out a pan and combine the salt, water, and barley inside. Bring this to a boil.
2. Cover the pot and reduce the heat to low. After 25 minutes of simmering, the water should be absorbed.
3. Divide the barley into six containers or jars. Divide the cherries in each and pour half a cup of the milk. Add in some almonds to each one too.
4. Close the jars tightly. Store in the fridge for five days or serve right away.

Sweet Potato Hash

What's inside:

Pepper
Salt

Black beans (1 can)
Dried oregano (1 tsp.)
Ground cumin (2 tsp.)
Sweet potato, diced (1)
Minced garlic (2 tsp.)
Diced yellow onion (1)
Olive oil (1 tsp.)

How to make:

1. Take out a skillet and add the oil inside. Add in the garlic and onion to cook for a few minutes.
2. Add in the oregano, cumin, and sweet potato. Cook another five minutes.
3. Place the lid on the skillet and reduce the heat to low. Let this cook together.
4. After fifteen minutes, increase the heat and add in the pepper, salt, and black beans. Let these warm up.
5. After five more minutes, divide between 6 containers and serve or store.

Green Smoothie

What's inside:

Plant based milk (4 c.)
Spinach (4 c.)
Hulled strawberries (4 c.)
Peeled bananas (4)

How to make:

1. Take out four freezer bags, quart sized. In each one, layer one banana (sliced or halved), one cup of strawberries, and one cup of spinach.
2. Seal and leave in freezer until needed.
3. To serve, take the frozen bag out of the freezer and place into a blender. Add one cup of milk for each serving and blend until smooth.

Smoothie Breakfast Bowl

What's inside:

Plant-based milk (4 c.)
Slivered almonds (.5 c.)
Fresh berries (2 c.)
Baked granola (1 c.)
Dragon fruit (1 c.)
Peeled bananas (4)

How to make:

1. Take out four freezer bags and layer in one sliced banana and .25 cup of dragon fruit. Put in the freezer.
2. Take out four small jelly jars and layer in the following in order: granola, berries, and almonds. Divide up evenly.
3. To starve, take out the fruit and add to a blender. Add in a cup of milk for each serving.

4. When smooth, pour into a bowl and add the contents of one prepared jar on top. Serve right away.

Tortilla Breakfast Casserole

What's inside

Shredded vegan Cheddar cheese (.5 c.)
Corn tortillas (10)
Hot sauce (2 tsp.)
Nutritional yeast (.25 c.)
Black beans (1 can)
Tofu spinach scramble (2 c.)
Cooking spray

How to make

1. Turn on the oven to 350 degrees. Use the cooking spray to prepare a baking pan.

2. Bring out a big bowl to combine the black beans, tofu scramble, hot sauce, and nutritional yeast.
3. Place five tortillas on the bottom of your baking pan. Spread half of your tofu and beans on and top with some cheese. Repeat, ending with the cheese on top.
4. Add to the oven. After 20 minutes, the dish is done. Take out of the oven and divide between six containers or serve.

Lunch

Green Pea Risotto

What's inside:

Pepper
Green peas (2 c.)
Nutritional yeast (2 tbsp.)
Lemon juice (3 tbsp.)
Salt (.25 tsp.)
Vegetable broth (2 c.)
Arborio rice (1 c.)
Minced garlic (4 tsp.)
Vegan butter (1 tsp.)

How to make:

1. Add the butter to a skillet and heat up. Then cook the garlic for three minutes.

2. Add the salt, broth, and rice. Bring this mixture to a boil while stirring and then reduce the heat. Allow to simmer for half an hour to make rice tender.
3. Now add in the lemon juice and nutritional yeast before folding in the peas. Taste before seasoning.
4. Divide between four single-serving containers and either store or serve right away.

Yummy Potatoes and Kale

What's inside:

Pepper
Great northern beans (1 can)
Kale (6 oz.)
Vegetable broth (.5 c.)
Salt
Russet potatoes (2)

How to make:

1. Wash the potatoes and dice them. Add into a pot with water and bring to a boil.
2. Cover the pot and let the potatoes cook. After twenty minutes, the potatoes will be tender and you can drain them out.
3. Pour the vegetable broth on top of these and add in the beans and kale. Cover the pot again and cook on a low heat to get the kale to turn bright green.

4. Using your potato masher, mash these ingredients together and season with some pepper and salt.
5. Divide the beans, kale, and potatoes between four containers and then serve or store.

Warm Vegetable Salad

What's inside:

Cashew cream (1 c.)
Pepper
Dried dill (2 tsp.)
Lime juice (2 tbsp.)
Olive oil (1 tbsp.)
Sliced carrots (1 lb.)
Quartered red potatoes (4)
Salt

How to make:

1. Fill up a big pot with some water and add the salt to it. Place the potatoes inside and let cook.
2. After eight minutes, add in the carrots and continue cooking. Another eight minutes will pass and both vegetables will become crisp and tender.
3. Drain the water out and return to the pot. Add in the salt, pepper, dill, lime juice, and olive oil and stir to coat.
4. Divide these among four containers or jars and spoon a bit of the cream on top. Serve or seal up.

Not Tuna Salad

What's inside:

Pepper (.25 tsp.)
Salt (.5 tsp.)

Vegan mayo (.25 c.)

Diced celery (.5 c.)

Chopped white onion (.5 c.)

Hearts of palm (1 can)

Chickpeas (1 can)

How to make:

1. Place the chickpeas into a bowl and mash them up roughly. Then add in the pepper, salt, mayo, celery, onion, and hearts of palm to make it creamy.
2. Add ¾ cup of the salad to four serving containers. Seal up and store or serve right away.

Red Bean and Corn Salad

What's inside:

Chopped Romaine lettuce (8 c.)

Barley, cooked (1 c.)

Corn (2 c.)

Kidney beans (2 cans)

Chili powder (1 tsp.)

Cashew cream (.25 c.)

How to make:

1. Set up four quart jars. Then bring out a bowl and whisk together the chili powder and cream. Pour a tablespoon of this into each jar.
2. Then divide up the kidney beans, corn, cooked barley, and romaine lettuce. Push it into the jar to fit. Add the lids on tightly.
3. Store these for up to five days.

Mediterranean Beans with Greens

What's inside:

Lemon juice (.5 c.)

Arugula (10 oz.)

Minced garlic (4 tsp.)

Olive oil (1 tsp.)

Vegetable broth (.5 c.)

Diced green olives (.25 c.)

Cannellini beans (2 cans)

Diced tomatoes (1 can).

How to make:

1. Bring out a pot and add in the beans, tomatoes, broth and olives inside. Bring to a boil and then reduce the heat to a simmer. This will take ten minutes.
2. Bring out a skillet and heat up the oil. Add in the garlic and let it brown. Add in the lemon and arugula and cook on a low heat for a few minutes.
3. After three minutes, divide the arugula among four containers and spoon the bean mixture on top before serving or storing.

Cheesy Polenta

What's inside:

Lemon juice (1 tbsp.)
Vegan butter (2 tsp.)
Nutritional yeast (.25 c.)
Chopped mushrooms (2 c.)
Olive oil (1 tsp.)
Ground turmeric (.5 tsp.)
Ground cumin (1 tsp.)
Salt (1 tsp.)
Cornmeal (1.75 c.)
Water (2 c.)
Vegetable broth (4 c.)

How to make:

1. Take out a pot and bring the water and broth to a boil. Slowly whisk the cornmeal in along with the turmeric, cumin, and salt.

2. Reduce the heat to low and cook to make it thicken. After fifteen minutes this will be done.
3. Bring out a pan and heat up the oil. Add the mushrooms and let it cook for a bit. After five minutes, set aside.
4. Add the polenta to a bowl and add in the mushrooms, lemon juice, butter, and nutritional yeast.
5. Divide this among six containers and let it cool before storing.

DINNER

Chickpea Salad

What's inside:

Olive oil (2 tbsp.)
Lemon juice (2 tbsp.)
Agave nectar (1 tbsp.)
Chopped parsley (.5 c.)
Pomegranate seeds (.5 c.)
Chickpeas (2 c.)
Cooked couscous (1 c.)

How to make

1. Bring out a big salad bowl and mix all of the ingredients together.
2. Serve as a salad, in a wrap, or add some salad greens to get some more protein.

Warm Quinoa Salad

What's inside:

Tahini (.33 c.)
Dry quinoa (2 c.)
Pepper
Salt
Water (4 c.)
Juiced lemon (1)
Garlic head (1)
Pomegranate seeds (.5 c.)

How to make:

1. Peel the outer layer off the head of garlic and then chop this top off so that the cloves are exposed.
2. Drizzle this with some oil and roast inside the oven for a bit. It will take about half an hour.

3. While those are cooking, add the quinoa and the water to a pot on the stove. Let this simmer.
4. After 15 minutes, the water should evaporate. When both are done cooking, peel the garlic and add it to your quinoa.
5. Add in the pomegranate, lemon juice, and tahini. Stir together.
6. Serve with some mixed greens and enjoy.

Black Bean Soup

What's inside:

Juiced lime (1)
Hot sauce
Ground cumin (1 tsp.)
Vegetable broth (1 c.)
Black beans (1 can)

How to make:

1. Bring out a big pot and add to the stove. Place all of the ingredients into it.
2. Let this mixture come to a boil and heat up. After half an hour, the soup should be done.
3. Add on the toppings that you would like and then serve!

Pineapple Quinoa Salad

What's inside:

Olive oil (2 tbsp.)
Diced cucumber (1)
Cilantro (.33 c.)
Mixed greens (4 c.)
Cooked quinoa (3 c.)
Diced pineapple (1 c.)

How to make:

1. Take out the pineapple and dice up a cup of it. Save the juice from this for later. Dice up the cucumber as well.
2. Toss the mixed greens into a bowl along with the pineapple juice, some salt, and olive oil.
3. In another bowl, mix together the cucumber, quinoa, and pineapple. Serve this on top of the mixed greens and enjoy.

Butternut Squash Gnocchi

What's inside:

Olive oil (2 tbsp.)
Salt
Basil (.25 c.)
Gnocchi (3 c.)
Vegetable broth (1 .)

Garlic cloves (3)

Diced butternut squash (.5)

How to make:

1. Slice and dice up one half of the squash. Add it to a pot with some olive oil. Allow it to cook until it is nice and tender.
2. After 30 minutes, add in the gnocchi and the vegetable broth to this. Bring it to a boil, and then reduce the mixture to a simmer.
3. Cook for a few minutes. As you stir, you should notice that the squash starts to break down to make a creamy sauce.
4. Now add in some vegan butter and basil and stir together. Remove this when the gnocchi is cooked through and you can serve.

No Cook Quesadilla

What's inside:

Lime wedges to serve
Fresh salsa (1 c.)
Tortillas (2)
Diced red onion .25)
Vegan queso (1 c.)
Avocado (1)

How to make

1. Take the tortilla and microwave for a minute. While that is going on, slice up the avocado in half and dice up your onions.
2. Add as much queso and avocado onto the tortillas as you would like and sprinkle with the onions.

3. When you are done, fold up the tortillas and serve with lime wedges and salsa for dipping.

BBQ Sandwich

What's inside:

Olive oil (1 tbsp.)
Shredded carrot (1)
Buns (92)
Vegan BBQ sauce (.5 c.)
Chickpeas (1 c.)
Tofu (1 block)

How to make:

1. Crumble up the tofu into the sizes you would like. Then add it to a pan with some olive oil and fry for a bit.
2. After the tofu reaches the consistency that you would like, add the chickpeas

into the pan and allow them to get warm.
3. Add in the BBQ sauce and stir to coat and warm up. Then take off the heat.
4. Lay out your buns and add this mixture on top. Top it all with some shredded carrots before serving.

SNACKS AND DESSERT

Risotto Bites

What's inside:

Green pea risotto (1.5 c.)
Chipotle powder (1 tsp.)
Paprika (1 tsp.)
Panko bread crumbs (.5 c.)

How to make:

1. Let the oven heat up to 425 degrees. Add some parchment paper to a baking sheet.
2. Take out a plate and combine the chipotle powder, paprika, and panko. Set to the side.

3. Roll two tablespoons of the risotto into a ball. Roll in the bread crumbs and add to the baking sheet. Do this 12 times.
4. Add to the oven to bake. After 15 minutes, they are done and you can take them out.
5. Cool down completely before storing in an airtight container.

Kale Chips

What's inside:

Salt (.25 tsp.)
Smoked paprika (.5 tsp.)
Chipotle powder (.5 tsp.)
Olive oil (1 tbsp.)
Kale (1 bunch)

How to make:

1. Turn on the oven and let it heat up to 275 degrees. Use some parchment paper to line a baking sheet.
2. Take out a bowl and tear up the kale. Add in the salt, smoked paprika, chipotle powder, and olive oil. Toss the kale around.
3. Add this to the prepared baking sheet in a single layer. Add to the oven to bake.
4. After 25 minutes, the chips are done. Take out of the oven and cool before serving.

Taco Pita Pizzas

What's inside:

Minced jalapeno (1 tsp.)
Chopped mushrooms (1 c.)
Pizza sauce (1 c.)
Refried beans, vegetarian (1 c.)
Pita bread pieces (4)

How to make:

1. Heat up the oven to 400 degrees. Line a baking sheet.
2. Assemble the pizzas. Lay out the pita pieces and add the beans, pizza sauce, and mushrooms on top.
3. Top with the jalapeno and then place onto the baking sheets and into the oven.
4. After seven minutes, take these out of the oven and let them cool down before serving.

Seed Crackers

What's inside

Water (.5 c.)
Dried oregano (.5 tsp.)
Cayenne pepper (.5 tsp.)

Vegan Worcestershire sauce (1 tsp.)

Tamari sauce (1 tsp.)

Minced garlic (1 tsp.)

Chia seeds (.25 c.)

Sesame seeds (.5 c.)

Sunflower seeds (.5 c.)

Pumpkin seeds (.75 c.)

How to make:

1. Turn on the oven and let it heat up to 325 degrees.
2. Inside a bowl, combine the water, oregano, cayenne, Worcestershire sauce, tamari, garlic, chia seeds, sesame seeds, sunflower seeds, and pumpkin seeds.
3. Add this to a baking sheet and spread out. Place the baking sheet into the oven to bake.

4. After 25 minutes, take the pan out of the oven and flip these over to have the wet side go up. Place back into the oven.
5. After another 20 minutes, take the dish out. Cool this down completely and then break into 20 pieces. Divide into four servings and enjoy.

Tamari Almonds

What's inside

Chili powder (2 tsp.)
Nutritional yeast (1 tbsp.)
Olive oil (2 tbsp.)
Tamari sauce (3 tbsp.)
Raw almonds (1 lb.)

How to make

1. Turn on the oven to 400 degrees.

2. Bring out a bowl and combine the olive oil, tamari, and almonds until well coated. Spread out onto a baking sheet and then place in the oven.
3. After ten minutes, take the almonds out of the oven and let them cool down a bit.
4. Season with chili powder and nutritional yeast. Move this over to a glass jar and then seal.

Roasted Chickpeas

What's inside:

Garlic powder (1 tsp.)
Smoked paprika (1 tsp.)
Olive oil (1 tsp.)
Chickpeas (1 can)

How to make:

1. Start this recipe by turning on the oven and letting it heat up to 425 degrees.

2. After you drain the chickpeas, pat them dry with a paper towel and move to a bowl. Add in the garlic powder, paprika, and oil.
3. Use a spoon or your hands to toss and coat. Spread out onto a baking sheet in a single layer. Add to the oven.
4. After 30 minutes, the chickpeas are done. Turn off the oven and leave the door open a bit.
5. Let these cool down in the oven. Transfer to a glass pint jar and serve when ready.

Veggie Pinwheels

What's inside:

Shredded carrots (.75 c.)
Edamame Hummus (.75 c.)
Swiss chard leaves (3)
Tortillas (3)

How to make:

1. Lay out one of the tortillas on a cutting board. Place a leaf of Swiss chard on top and then spread some hummus on top. Top with the carrots.
2. Start at one end of the tortilla and start to roll tightly to the other side. When that is done, slice into 6 parts.
3. Add these parts to a storage container and then repeat with the rest of the tortillas to finish.

Chapter 9: Week Two Meal Plan and Grocery List

The Meal Plan

Day 1:	Day 2:	Day 3	Day 4
Breakfast: Tofu and Spinach Scramble Lunch: TLT Wraps Dinner Cauliflower Sheet Pan Snack: Baked Granola	Breakfast: Easy Pancakes Lunch: Chili Dinner: Mediterranean Quesadilla Snack: Banana Nut Bread Bars	Breakfast: Key Lime Smoothie Bowl Lunch: Quinoa Pilaf Dinner: Cauliflower Nachos Snack: Chocolate Truffles	Breakfast: Gluten Free Pancakes Lunch: Quinoa and Kale Bowls Dinner: Simple Pasta Snack: Minty Fruit

			Salad
Day 5	Day 6:	Day 7:	
Breakfast: French Toast Lunch: Asian Chili Dinner: Sweet and Savory Tofu Snack: Energy Bites	Breakfast: Tofu Scramble Lunch: Cucumber Salad Dinner: Pumpkin Curry Snack: Black Bean Brownies	Breakfast: Loaded Toast Lunch: Vegan Mac and Cheese Dinner: Stuffed zucchini Boats Snack: Roasted Apple Bites	

The Grocery List

½ c. apple cider	¾ c. dry white wine	4 slices whole grain bread
2 tortillas	2 Tbsp. agave nectar	4 Tbsp. baking powder
1 tsp. baking soda	1 c. carob chips	1 c. Cocoa powder
3 Tbsp. Vanilla	2 c. oat flour	1 c. whole wheat flour
2 Tbsp. sesame seeds	2 tsp. vegan sugar	1 c. brown sugar
1.25 c. maple syrup	4 Tbsp. nutritional yeast	3 Tbsp. key lime juice
1 c. gluten free oats	5 c. rolled oats	3 cans black beans
3 cans chickpeas	½ c. black olives	1 ½ c. pumpkin
½ c. guacamole	¼ c. hummus	4 ½ c. vegetable broth

1 can coconut milk	1 c. almond butter	¼ c. tahini
½ c. diced tomatoes	2 tsp. tomato paste	1 c. TVP
1 c. vegan cheddar cheese	¼ c. vegan parmesan	¼ tsp. liquid smoke
½ c. vegan mayo	1 tsp. mustard	4 Tbsp. coconut oil
12 Tbsp. Olive oil	Cooking spray	2 c. salsa
1 tsp. Vegan Worcestershire	1/3 c. white wine vinegar	¼ c. sunflower seed butter
3 Tbsp. vegan butter	3 flax eggs	1 c. oat milk
1/3 c. plant based milk	3 tsp. chili powder	1 tsp. chipotle powder
½ tsp. red pepper flakes	4 tbsp. cinnamon	2 tsp. cumin
¼ c. curry powder	1 tbsp. dill	1 tsp. garlic powder
1 tsp. garlic salt	8 mint leaves	1 tsp. onion powder
1 tsp. paprika	½ tsp. parsley	Pepper

Salt	¼ tsp. thyme	¾ turmeric
2 c. millet	3 ½ quinoa	8 oz. Elbow
6 oz. spaghetti	4 apples	1 avocado
3 bananas	1 pepper	1 c. blueberries
3 carrots	3 heads of cauliflower	3 celery stalks
1 c. coconut	2 c. cucumber	1 eggplant
12 garlic cloves	1 head of garlic	2 c. greens
6 oz. kale	1 lemon	¾ c. lemon juice
8 lettuce leaves	4 c. shredded lettuce	½ c. mushrooms
2 c. onion	2 c. sweet onion	¾ c. red onion
1 yellow onion	1 red pepper	2 Tbsp. jalapeno
2 c. pineapple	2 c. raspberries	5 ½ c. spinach
2 c. strawberries	3 tomatoes	4 zucchini
1 can diced tomatoes	Cherry tomatoes	1 roll vegan biscuit dough
1 lb. tempeh	1 c tofu	3 blocks tofu

¾ c. pitted dates	1 c. dried fruit	1 c. cashews
1 ½ c. chopped walnuts	¼ c. pumpkin seeds	4 vegan tortillas

The Recipes

BREAKFAST

Tofu and Spinach Scramble

What's inside:

Spinach (5 c.)

Pepper (.25 tsp.)

Salt (.5 tsp.)

Ground turmeric (.5 tsp.)

Ground cumin (.5 tsp.)

Chili powder (1 tsp.)

Chopped carrots (2)

Chopped celery stalks (3)

Minced garlic (3 tsp.)

Diced yellow onion (1)

Olive oil (1 tsp.)

Tofu (1 package)

How to make:

1. Press and drain out the tofu by placing it wrapped up on a towel and over the sink. Place the cutting board on tofu and then a can on top. Remove after ten minutes.
2. Crumble the tofu with a potato masher in a bowl and set aside.
3. Heat up some oil in a skillet. Cook the carrots, celery, garlic, and onion for a few minutes.
4. When the onion is soft, add in the pepper, salt, turmeric, cumin, chili powder, and tofu.
5. After 8 more minutes, add the spinach. Cover the skillet and turn down the heat.
6. Let the spinach steam and then divide up into 5 servings.

Easy Pancakes

What's inside:

Packed greens (2 c.)
Chopped onion (.5 c.)
Chopped mushrooms (.5 c.)
Olive oil (2 tbsp.)
Lemon juice (.25 c.)
Unsweetened plant-based milk (.33 c.)
Crumbled tofu (1 c.)
Salt (.25 tsp.)
Baking soda (.5 tsp.)
Onion powder (1 tsp.)
Garlic salt (1 tsp.)
Whole wheat flour (1 c.)

How to make:

1. Using a big bowl, combine the salt, baking soda, onion powder, garlic salt, and flour.

2. Use your blender to mix the olive oil, lemon juice, milk, and tofu. Puree on high speed for half a minute.
3. Add the blended ingredients into the bowl and whisk to combine well. Gently fold in the greens, mushrooms, and onion.
4. Prepare a skillet and heat it up. Add half a cup of batter for each pancake.
5. Cook until some bubbles start to form and then flip the pancakes over to finish. Repeat with the rest of the batter.
6. Divide into four servings and enjoy.

Gluten Free Pancakes

What's inside:

Salt (1 tsp.)
Flax eggs (2)
Oat milk (1 c.)
Vanilla (2 tbsp.)

Baking powder (2 tbsp.)
Oat flour (2 c.)

How to make:

1. Take out a bowl and mix together the baking powder and oat flour. Use a second bowl to whisk together the egg and the oat milk. Mix the two bowls together.
2. Warm up some cooking oil in a frying pan. Add .25 cup of batter onto the skillet and let it make a pancake.
3. When you see some bubbles through the batter, use the spatula to flip the pancakes once.
4. Repeat with the rest of the batter and serve with some cinnamon or syrup.

Key Lime Pie Smoothie Bowl

What's inside:

Agave nectar (2 tbsp.)
Granny Smith apple (1)
Spinach (.5 c.)
Banana (1)
Key lime juice (3 tbsp.)

How to make:

1. Take out a blender and add the banana in it. Blend on a low setting.
2. Add in a tablespoon of water at a time and blend until the banana has a creamy consistency.
3. Add in the remainder of the ingredients and blend to make it creamy and smooth.

French Toast

What's inside:

Vanilla (1 tsp.)
Cinnamon (1 tsp.)
Maple syrup (3 tbsp.)
Coconut milk (1 c.)
Bread slices (4)

How to make:

1. Bring out a bowl and mix together the maple syrup, vanilla, cinnamon, and coconut milk.
2. Take each slice of bread and soak it in the mixture, coating both sides completely.
3. Take out a skillet and warm it up on the stove. Add each bread slice to the skillet and cook to make both sides nice and golden brown.

4. Add any of the additional syrup over the cooked slices and enjoy.

Tofu Scramble

What's inside:

Salt (1 tsp.)
Garlic powder (1 tsp.)
Diced onion (.25)
Nutritional yeast (2 tbsp.)
Turmeric (.25 tsp.)
Tofu (1 block)

How to make:

1. Bring out a bowl and break up the tofu into it. Heat up the oil in a frying pan and then add in the tofu.
2. After five minutes of cooking the tofu, add in the turmeric, garlic powder,

onion, and nutritional yeast. Coat the tofu with this mixture.

3. Allow this to cook for a bit longer. To get a texture like scrambled eggs, cook for 10 minutes. Never go above 15 minutes.

Loaded Toast

What's inside:

Red onion (.25 c.)
Diced tomatoes (.5 c.)
Sunflower seed butter (.25 c.)
Avocado (1)
Whole grain bread (4 slices)

How to make:

1. Bring out a bowl and add the diced onion, salt, and pepper inside along with the mashed avocado.
2. Dice up the tomato and add to a bowl.

3. If you would like this to be warm, toast up the bread as you work with the veggies.
4. Spread a bit of butter on each slice and then spread on the avocado mixture. Top with the tomatoes and serve.

LUNCH

TLT Wraps

What's inside:

Vegan mayo (.5 c.)
Tomatoes (2)
Lettuce leaves (8)
Vegan tortilla (4)
Cayenne pepper (1 tsp.)
Liquid smoke (.25 tsp.)
Vegan Worcestershire sauce (1 tsp.)
Olive oil (2 tsp.)
Maple syrup (.25 c.)
Tempeh (1 lb.)
Water (1 c.)

How to make

1. Boil some water on the stove. Add a steamer basket on top with the tempeh inside. Cover and steam.
2. After ten minutes, remove the tempeh and let it cool before slicing into 16 parts.
3. Bring out a small bowl and whisk together the cayenne pepper, liquid smoke, Worcestershire sauce, olive oil, and maple syrup.
4. Add some cooking spray to a skillet and warm up. Add the tempeh strips and pour the sauce on top. Turn around halfway through cooking.
5. After 6 minutes, move the tempeh to a plate.
6. To assemble these, have one tortilla, two leaves of lettuce, two tomato slices, four tempeh strips, and two tablespoons of mayo.

7. Roll up and store or eat right away.

Chili

What's inside

Diced jalapeno pepper (2 tbsp.)

Tomato paste (2 tsp)

Diced tomatoes (1 can)

Black beans (1 can)

Red pepper flakes (.5 tsp.)

Ground cumin (1 tsp.)

Chili powder (1 tsp.)

Paprika (1 tsp.)

Chipotle powder (1 tsp)

Minced garlic (3 tsp.)

Diced onion (1 c.)

Olive oil (1 tbsp.)

No-beef broth (1.5 c.)

Textured vegetable protein TVP (1 c.)

Pepper

Salt

How to make:

1. Bring out a bowl and combine a cup of warm broth with the TVP. Let it stand for ten minutes.
2. Heat up the oil in a big pot. Add the garlic and onion and cook for a few minutes.
3. Add in the TVP, red pepper flakes, cumin, chili powder, paprika, and chipotle pepper. Stir well.
4. Add in the rest of the broth, the jalapeno, tomato paste, tomatoes, and black beans. Bring this to a boil.
5. Cover the pot and reduce heat. Simmer the ingredients for 20 minutes.
6. Divide this between four containers and serve.

Quinoa Pilaf

What's inside:

Chopped walnuts (.5 c.)
Salt (.5 tsp.)
Dried thyme (.5 tsp.)
Dried parsley (.5 tsp.)
Vegetable broth (1.5 c.)
Diced carrot (1 c.)
Chopped red onion (.5 c.)
Olive oil (1 tsp.)
Dry Quinoa (1 c.)

How to make:

1. Rinse off the quinoa. Bring out a saucepan to heat up the oil. Add in the carrot and onion and cook for a few minutes.

2. Now add in the quinoa, salt, thyme, parsley, and broth. Bring to a boil. Cover the pan and let it simmer for a bit.
3. After 15 minutes, take the pan from the stove and set to the side. Fluff before adding in the walnuts.
4. Divide a cup of the quinoa into four containers and either serve or save for later.

Quinoa and Kale Bowls

What's inside:

Pepper
Salt
Lemon juice (3 tsp.)
Chopped tomato (1)
Chopped kale (6 oz.)
Water (2 c.)
Rinsed quinoa, dry (1 c.)

How to make:

1. Combine the water and quinoa in a pot and bring to a boil. Cover and let simmer. After fifteen minutes, take from the heat and add in the kale. Set to the side.
2. After five minutes, add the pepper, salt, lemon juice, and tomato.
3. Divide this up into four storage containers and then serve or store for later.

Asian Chili

What's inside:

Hot sauce (1 tbsp.)
Hot water (2 tbsp.)
Red miso paste (2 tbsp.)
Vegetable broth (2 c.)
Diced tomatoes (1 can)

Red beans (1 can)

Green cabbage (2 c.)

Chopped carrots (1 c.)

Minced garlic (3 tsp.)

Diced onion (1 c.)

Sesame oil (1 tsp.)

Tamari sauce (2 tsp.)

How to make

1. Bring out a pot and heat the oil. Add in the carrot, garlic, and onion to cook until they become translucent.
2. Add in the broth, tomatoes, beans, and cabbage. Stir around and bring to a boil.
3. Cover the pot and turn to low heat. Allow to simmer. Mix together the hot water and the miso paste while this is cooking and set aside.
4. After fifteen minutes are up, remove the chili and add in the hot sauce and miso mixture. Add in the tamari.

5. Divide the chili up into four glass jars and let it cool before sealing.

Cucumber Quinoa Salad

What's inside

Shredded lettuce (4 c.)
Diced cucumber (2 c.)
Sliced sweet onions (2 c.)
Pepper
Salt
Vegan sugar (1.5 tsp.)
Chopped dill (1 tbsp.)
Olive oil (2 tbsp.)
White wine vinegar (.33 c.)
Water (2.25 c.)
Dry Quinoa (1.5 c.)

How to make

1. Take out a pot and combine the water and quinoa. Boil and cook for 15 minutes.
2. Take the pot from the stove and let it have a few minutes to stand. Then fluff with a fork.
3. While that is cooking, combine the pepper, salt, sugar, dill, olive oil, and vinegar.
4. Into some jars, add a few tablespoons of the dressing, some onions, cucumber, quinoa, and lettuce. Seal and store.

Vegan Mac and Cheese

What's inside:

Lemon juice (2 tsp.)
Nutritional yeast (2 tbsp.)
Minced garlic (2 tsp.)
Vegan elbow macaroni (8 oz.)
Salt for the water

How to make:

1. Bring out a pot of salted water and let it boil. Add in the pasta and cook according to the directions on the package.
2. Add in the Kale, lemon juice, nutritional yeast, and garlic. Stir to combine well.
3. Divide the mac and cheese between four glass jars. Allow time to cool before sealing.

DINNER

Cauliflower Sheet Pan

What's inside:

Olive oil (2 tbsp.)
Lemon juiced (1)
Salt
Tahini (.25 c.)
Canned chickpeas (1 c.)
Garlic head (1)
Cauliflower (1 head)

How to make:

1. Turn on the oven and let it heat up to 350 degrees. Chop your cauliflower and drizzle with some oil.

2. Cut the tops from the garlic and leave the cloves open. Drizzle with the oil and sprinkle on some salt.
3. Add both the cauliflower and the garlic onto a pan and bake. After 35 minutes, you can take them out of the oven and let them cool down.
4. Squeeze the garlic out and get rid of the skin. Bring out a bowl and mix together the garlic, cauliflower, salt, chickpeas, lemon juice, and tahini.
5. Serve with some tortillas and guacamole if you choose.

Mediterranean Quesadilla

What's inside:

Salt
Olive oil
Cherry tomatoes
Tortillas (2)

Sliced red pepper, roasted (1)
Sliced eggplant, roasted (1)
Garlic hummus .25 c)

How to make:

1. Add some oil and salt to the eggplant slices and move to a baking tray. Slice the red pepper and add as well.
2. Turn on the oven and let it heat up to 400 degrees. Add the baking tray inside to cook.
3. After 30 minutes, the vegetables are done and you can take them out.
4. Heat up your tortillas for a minute on each side. Spread out some hummus on the tortillas and add the red pepper slices and eggplant on top.
5. Drizzle on some oil and the tomatoes and then serve.

Cauliflower Nachos

What's inside:

Guacamole (.5 c.)
Salsa (.5 c.)
Black beans (1 can)
Vegan cheddar cheese (1 c.)
Cauliflower head (1)

How to make:

1. Take the cauliflower and chop it into florets. Drizzle on some olive oil.
2. Turn the oven on and let it heat up to 400 degrees for a bit. You want to turn this slightly brown.
3. Take the pan out of the oven after 25 minutes. Cover this in black beans and vegan cheese. Add to the oven to melt the cheese.

4. Serve this with some guacamole and salsa when ready.

Simple Pasta

What's inside:

Salt (1 tsp.)
Olive oil (2 tbsp.)
Vegetable broth (1.5 c.)
Minced garlic cloves (4)
Vegan Parmesan (.25 c.)
Spaghetti (6 oz.)
Dry white wine (.75 c.)

How to make:

1. Bringout a pot and heat up the oil inside. Throw the minced garlic inside and cook for a few minutes before adding in the spaghetti, wine, and broth.

2. Cook this for a few minutes until the pasta is cooked through.
3. When the pasta is ready (there will be a bit of liquid left), you can add in the vegan parmesan and stir while it is still hot.

Sweet and Savory Tofu

What's inside

Pepper
Salt
Cooking oil (1 tbsp.)
Mustard (1 tsp.)
Maple syrup (3 tbsp.)
Apple cider (.5 c.)
Tofu, firm (1 block)

How to make:

1. Slice up the tofu going lengthwise to get the thickness that you want.
2. In a different bowl, whisk together the mustard, maple syrup, apple cider, and apple cider vinegar.
3. Dip the tofu into this, and coat on all sides. Add to a baking pan and turn the oven on to 400 degrees.
4. Bake the tofu for half an hour. Add on more of the reserved liquid if needed.
5. Serve this warm or cold in a salad or with some rice.

Pumpkin Curry

What's inside:

Water
Cauliflower (1 c.)
Curry powder (.25 c.)
Chickpeas (2 cans)
Coconut milk (1 can)

Cubed pumpkin (1.5 c.)

How to make:

1. Take out a big pot and add in the cauliflower, pumpkin, salt, curry powder, and coconut milk together.
2. Bring all of this to a boil before reducing to a simmer. Add in some more water as needed.
3. When the pumpkin is cooked to the right consistency, bring out the immersion blender and make this a creamy base.
4. Add in the chickpeas and allow them to heat up before serving.

Stuffed Zucchini Boats

What's inside:

Pepper

Salt

Diced bell pepper (1)

Sliced black olives (.5 c.)

Cooked millet (2 c.)

Salsa (1.5 c.)

Zucchinis (4)

How to make:

1. Turn on the oven and let it heat up to 375 degrees. As the oven heats up, cut off the ends of the zucchini and slice in half.
2. Use a spoon to take out the pulp and leave some room to pack the zucchini full of things.
3. Add the zucchini onto a baking pan and add to the oven. After 20 minutes, take the zucchini out of the oven and drain out the water.

4. Bring out a bowl and mix together the pepper, salt, diced bell peppers, salsa, black olives, and millet.
5. Use this mixture to pack your zucchini and place back into the oven. After 15 minutes, the zucchini should be done and you can serve.

SNACKS AND DESSERTS

Baked Granola

What's inside:

Salt
Olive oil (2 tbsp.)
Maple syrup (.25 c.)
Sesame seeds (2 tbsp.)
Pumpkin seeds (.25 c.)
Chopped nuts (.5 c.)
Dried fruit (1 c.)
Rolled oats (3 c.)

How to make:

1. Turn on the oven and let it heat up to 300 degrees.
2. While the oven heats up, bring out a bowl and combine the salt, coconut oil,

maple syrup, sesame seeds, pumpkin seeds, nuts, fruit, and oats. Toss to coat.
3. Add this to a baking sheet and spread out evenly. Add to the oven and let it bake.
4. After 30 minutes, take this out of the oven and allow to cool. Then transfer it to six single serving storage containers and store.

Banana Nut Bread Bars

What's inside

Chopped walnuts (.25 c.)
Salt
Old-fashioned rolled oats (2 c.)
Vanilla (.5 tsp.)
Maple syrup (1 tbsp.)
Ripe bananas (2)
Cooking spray

How to make:

1. Turn on the oven and let it heat up to 350 degrees. Set up a baking pan with some cooking spray.
2. Bring out a bowl and use a fork to mash the bananas. Add the vanilla and maple syrup. Mix well before adding the walnuts, salt, and oats.
3. Move this batter into the baking pan and add into the oven. After 25 minutes the bars should be done.
4. Cool these down a bit and then serve or store for later.

Chocolate Truffles

What's inside:

Cocoa powder (2 tbsp.)
Shredded coconut (1 c.)

Coconut oil (2 tbsp.)

Pitted dates (.75 c.)

Raw cashews (1 c.)

How to make:

1. Take out the food processor and combine the cocoa powder, .5 cup of shredded coconut, coconut oil, dates, and cashews.
2. Pulse these to make a cookie dough. Spread the rest of the coconut on a plate.
3. Form the mixture into some balls and roll over the coconut to cover. Add to a baking sheet and repeat with 12 truffles.
4. Place in the fridge to set for an hour or more before serving.

Minty Fruit Salad

What's inside

Mint leaves (8)

Blueberries (1 c.)

Raspberries (2 c.)

Chopped strawberries (2 c.)

Chopped pineapple (2 c.)

Maple syrup (4 tsp.)

Lemon juice (.25 c.)

How to make:

1. Bring out four Mason jars.
2. Split the ingredients up between them, starting with the lemon juice and ending with the mint leaves.
3. Close the jars tightly and then serve or store.

Energy Bites

What's inside:

Cinnamon (1 tsp.)

Gluten free oats (1 c.)

Carob chips (.66 c.)

Maple syrup (2 tbsp.)

Almond butter (.66 c.)

How to make

1. Bring out a big bowl and mix all of the ingredients together until well combined.
2. Place this bowl into the fridge and let it set for a bit.
3. After ten minutes, take the bowl out of the fridge and shape into some balls. Store in the fridge until you are ready to serve.

Black Bean Brownies

What's inside:

Coconut oil (2 tbsp.)

Salt (.25 tsp.)

Flax egg (1)

Cocoa powder (.75 c.)

Maple syrup (.5 c.)

Baking powder (2 tbsp.)

Cooked black beans (1.5 c.)

How to make:

1. Turn on the oven and let it heat up to 350 degrees.
2. Drain out the black beans and put in the food processor. Blend until smooth, adding in some more water as needed.
3. In a bowl, mix together the black beans with everything else. Add water so that you end up with a brownie-like batter.
4. Pour into a prepared pan and bake. After 30 minutes, these are all done and you can let them cool down and serve.

Roasted Apple Bites

What's inside:

Vegan biscuit dough (1 roll)
Brown sugar (.33 c.)
Melted vegan butter (3 tbsp.)
Cinnamon (3.5 tbsp.)
Apples (3)

How to make:

1. Bring out a bowl and combine the brown sugar with the melted butter and cinnamon.
2. Slice the apple into smaller pieces and dip each into the mix. Then wrap into the vegan biscuit dough.
3. Spread this out onto a baking sheet. Turn on the oven and let it heat up to 350 degrees.

4. Add the apple pieces into the oven and let them bake. After 15 minutes, take out and let them cool down before serving.

Chapter 10: Week Three Meal Plan and Grocery List

MEAL PLAN

Day 1:	Day 2:	Day 3:	Day 4
Breakfast: German Pancakes Lunch: Meatless Loaf Dinner: Quinoa Burger Snack: Bow Tie Chips	Breakfast: Banana French Toast Lunch: Tropical Protein Bowl Dinner: Hummus and Avocado Wrap Snack:	Breakfast: Protein Muffins Lunch: Rainbow Pinwheels Dinner: Avocado Sandwich Snack: Vegan Meatballs	Breakfast: Overnight Oats Lunch: Spaghetti Squash and Sauce Dinner: Fake Tuna Salad Snack: Bow Tie Chips

	Roasted Almonds		
Day 5: Breakfast: Tofu and Spinach Scramble Lunch: Simple Stir Fry Dinner: Salad and Falafel Sandwich Snack: Vegan Meatballs	Day 6: Breakfast: Breakfast Bowls Lunch: Asian Chili Dinner: BLT Sandwich Snack: Roasted Almonds	Day 7: Breakfast: Loaded Toast Lunch: Warm Vegetable Salad Dinner: BLT Sandwich Snack: Bow Tie Chips	

GROCERY LIST

2 slice pumpernickel bread	7 slices whole grain bread	2 pieces pita bread
2 corn tortillas	1 flour tortilla	1 tsp. baking powder
½ c. chocolate chips	½ tsp. vanilla	½ c. almond flour
1 c. whole wheat flour	1 Tbsp. almond meal	½ Tbsp. flaxseed meal
1 Tbsp. cornstarch	2 tsp. maple syrup	1 Tbsp. nutritional yeast
1 c. oats	1 can black beans	1 qt. garbanzo beans
½ c. hummus	1 c. green lentils	½ c. red lentils
10 pickle slices	2 scoops protein powder	1 c. applesauce
1 can cranberry	½ c. almond	1 c. tahini

sauce	butter	
½ c. sun dried tomatoes	½ c. Green goddess dressing	½ c. soy-tahini dressing
Thousand Island dressing	½ c. ketchup	2 tbsp. vegan mayo
1 tbsp. Dijon mustard	Mustard1	2 tbsp. olive oil
1 ½ c. BB sauce	1 tbsp. soy sauce	5 flax eggs
3 c. almond milk	½ c. sauerkraut	2 lbs. vegan meatballs
¼ c. basil	2 tsp. cinnamon	4 tbsp. garlic powder
1 tsp. paprika	Salt	Pepper
1 ½ tsp. Italian seasoning blend	¼ c. coconut bacon	3 c. quinoa
2 c. rice noodles	1 c. zucchini noodles	2 c. bow tie pasta
1/3 c. alfalfa sprouts	1 apple	1 c. arugula
¼ avocado	2 avocados	1 banana
3 bell peppers	2 carrots	½ c. celery

6 garlic cloves	1 c. greens	1 package Romain lettuce
1 mango	1 ½ c. onion	1 red onion
1 spaghetti squash	1 bunch spinach	3 tomatoes
2 c. almonds	½ c. cashews	7 falafel balls

The Recipes

BREAKFAST

German Pancakes

What's inside:

Flax eggs (3)
Salt (1 pinch)
Whole wheat flour (1 c.)
Almond milk (1 c.)
Applesauce (2 tbsp.)

How to make:

1. Turn on the air fryer and turn it on. As it heats up, set in a ramekin inside.
2. Take out a bowl and blend together all of the ingredients into a smooth batter. Add in small amounts of milk or

applesauce to thin it out if you think it is too thick.
3. Spray the ramekin and pour one serving of batter on it. Let this air fry for about six minutes. It may come out a bit hard, but it will soften when it cools down.
4. You can store these in the fridge and make a new serving each day, or keep repeating these steps in order to make a lot of pancakes for the day.
5. Add your favorite garnish and enjoy.

Banana French Toast

What's inside:

Cinnamon (.25 tsp.)
Wheat bread (5 slices)
Flaxseed meal (.5 tbsp.)
Vanilla (.5 tsp.)
Almond milk (1.25 c.)
Almond meal (1 tbsp.)

Banana (1)

How to make:

1. Take out a large and shallow bowl and then mash up the banana inside. Add in the cinnamon, almond milk, and flaxseed. Stir this in the batter.
2. Take out a skillet and let it heat up. Coat this with some coconut oil and heat up.
3. Take the pieces of bread and dip them into the batter. Press down a bit to make sure that the bread is fully coated on both sides.
4. Move to the griddle and cook to make a golden brown color. This takes a few minutes on both sides.
5. Add some of your favorite toppings to this and serve.

Protein Muffins

What's inside:

Almond flour (.5 c.)
Almond butter (.5 c.)
Applesauce (1 c.)
Baking powder (1 tsp.)
Chocolate chips (.5 c.0
Protein powder (2 scoops)

How to make:

1. Turn on the oven and give it time to heat up to 350 degrees. Take out a muffin tin and grease it up.
2. Take out a bowl and add in all of the dry ingredients. Then add in the almond butter and applesauce. Mix to combine before adding in the chocolate chips.
3. Divide this batter between the prepared muffin tins and then add to the oven.

After 15 minutes the muffins should be done.
4. Take the muffins out of the oven and give them time to cool down before serving.

Overnight Oats

What's inside:

Maple syrup (2 tsp.)
Chopped apple (1)
Old fashioned oats (.5 c.)
Cinnamon (1 tsp.)
Almond milk (.5 c.)

How to make:

1. Take out a jar and combine all of the ingredients inside.
2. Put the jar into the fridge overnight.

3. When you wake up, the oatmeal will be ready for you!

LUNCH

Meatless Loaf

What's inside:

Diced onion (1)
Ketchup (.25 c.)
Garlic powder (3 Tbsp.)
Oats (.5 c.)
Green lentils (1 c.)

How to make:

1. Add your lentils to a pot and cover them with water. Bring the water to a boil before reducing the heat and simmering.
2. After forty minutes, the lentils should be cooked through. Once they are done, set aside without draining so they can cool.

3. Use a food processor to blend half of your lentils up. Use a spoon to mix together the ketchup, oats, garlic powder, and onion.
4. Add to a bread pan and place into the oven at 350 degrees. After 45 minutes, you can take this out and serve warm.

Tropical Protein Bowl

What's inside:

Green goddess dressing (.25 c.)
Arugula (1 c.)
Diced mango (1 ripe)
Canned black beans (1 c.)
Cooked quinoa (2 c.)

How to make:

1. Rinse off the mixed greens and the black beans.

2. Bring out a few serving bowls and split the arugula between them. Top with the prepared quinoa and black beans.
3. Dice up the mango and add it on top. Top everything with the goddess dressing and pumpkin seeds and serve.

Rainbow Pinwheels

What's inside:

Mixed greens (1 c.)
Corn tortillas (2)
Hummus (.25 c.)
Sliced carrot (1)
Bell peppers (2)

How to make:

1. Slice up the bell peppers and carrots. Rinse off the mixed greens if needed.

2. Lay out the tortillas and slather the hummus on top of it.
3. Top this with the mixed greens and veggies, arranging in the pattern that you want.
4. Roll up the tortillas and then slice into four pieces each before serving.

Spaghetti Squash and Sauce

What's inside:

Cashews (.5 c.)
Chopped sun-dried tomatoes (.5 c.)
Basil (.25 c.)
Minced garlic cloves (3)
Spaghetti squash (1)

How to make:

1. Slice the spaghetti squash in half. Scoop the seeds out and throw them away or roast to use later.
2. Turn on the oven to 400 degrees. Add the squash inside and bake to make tender. It is going to be done in 40 minutes.
3. While this is cooking, bring out the food processor and combine the tomatoes, garlic, basil, and cashews together. Blend to make the consistency that you want.
4. When the squash is done, use a fork to scoop the insides out.
5. Mix this with the tomato sauce and then top with some vegan parmesan, salt or basil before serving.

Simple Stir Fry

What's inside:

Cooking oil (1 tbsp.)

Bell pepper (1 red)

Sliced carrot (1)

Zucchini noodles (1 c.)

Soy-tahini dressing (.25 c.)

Rice noodles (2 c.)

How to make:

1. Bring out a skillet and let the cooking oil heat up. When the oil is warm, add in the veggies and cook for a bit.
2. While the vegetables are cooking, bring some water to a boil. Add in the rice noodles and let them cook to become tender. This will be done in ten minutes.
3. When your vegetables are done the way you would like, toss them with the soy-tahini dressing and serve over the rice noodles.

DINNER

Quinoa Burgers

What's inside:

Salt (1 tsp.)
Dry Quinoa (1 c.)
Flax eggs (2)
Diced red onion (1)
Minced garlic cloves (3)
Dry red lentils (.5 c.)

How to make:

1. Bring out a pot and combine the three cups of water, quinoa, and lentils. Bring this to a boil and then reduce it to a simmer. Cook until the liquid is gone.
2. Now you can bring out a bowl and combine the onions, salt, garlic, and flax

egg together. When it is done, mix in the lentil and quinoa mixture.

3. Use your hands to shape this into burgers and put them on a baking sheet. Freeze if you want to save for later.
4. Turn on the oven to 400 degrees. Place the burgers inside to bake. After 20 minutes, turn them around and bake a bit longer. Serve warm.

Hummus with Avocado Wrap

What's inside:

Sliced avocado (.25)
Alfalfa sprouts (.33 c.)
Hummus (3 tbsp.)
Tomato slices (4)
Flour tortilla (1)

How to make:

1. Heat up the flour tortillas for about ten seconds in the microwave.
2. Spread out the hummus right down the center of the tortilla and then add the rest of the ingredients.
3. Wrap up the tortilla and then serve.

Avocado Sandwich

What's inside:

Thousand Island dressing
Mashed avocado (.5)
Mustard
Sauerkraut (.25 c.)
Pumpernickel bread (2 slices)

How to make:

1. Lay out both slices of bread. Spread out the Thousand Island dressing on one slice and the mustard on the other.

2. Add a bit of oil to a skillet and then put the dry sides of the bread down. Add the avocado to one slice and the sauerkraut on the other.
3. Grill these for a few minutes until the bread becomes browned and then put the two halves together before enjoying.

Fake Tuna Salad

What's inside

Chopped onion (.5 c.)
Salt
Chopped celery (.5 c.)
Vegan Mayo (2 tbsp.)
Cooked garbanzo beans (1 qt.)
Dijon mustard (1 tbsp.)

How to make:

1. Start this out by bringing out a big bowl and adding in all of the ingredients above to this bowl outside the mayo. Mix the ingredients and mash up the beans just a bit.
2. Add in enough of the vegan mayo to make the salad moist, just the way that you like it.
3. Serve this on some bread or on top of the lettuce.

Salad and Falafel Sandwich

What's inside

Dill pickle slices (10
Tahini (1 c.)
Sliced tomato 91)
Falafel balls (7)
Pita bread (2 pieces)
Stemmed spinach (1 bunch)

How to make:

1. Follow the instructions on the packaging of the falafel. Cook these all the way through to make them brown and crispy.
2. Take out the pita and add the spinach on top. Then crumble on top the falafel as well.
3. Add the dill pickles and the tomatoes to this as well and toss around.
4. Add a bit of the tahini on top before serving.

BLT Sandwich

What's inside

Coconut bacon (.25 c.)
Red tomato (1)
Salt
Pepper

Ripe avocado (1)
Romaine lettuce leaves
Whole grain bread (2 slices)
How to make:

1. Make up some coconut bacon ahead of time and freeze anything that is leftover for this.
2. Toast the bread to start. Halve your avocado and pit it. Scoop out the flesh and add to a bowl with some salt. Mash it up with a fork to get a smooth texture.
3. Spread this mashed avocado on both pieces of bread. Put some coconut bacon on one slice and press them down a bit.
4. Slice the tomato and place on top of the bacon slices.
5. Add the lettuce and then top with the other slice of bread before serving.

SNACKS

Bow Tie Chips

What's inside

Italian seasoning blend (1.5 tsp.)
Salt (.5 tsp.)
Nutritional yeast (1 tbsp.)
Bow tie pasta (2 c.)
Olive oil (1 tbsp.)

How to make

1. Start by cooking your pasta, but only do it for half the time that the package recommends.
2. Drain out the pasta and then add in the nutritional yeast, Italian seasoning, and olive oil. Toss these together.

3. Add this mixture to the air fryer. Cook for another 5 minutes with the air fryer at 390 degrees.
4. After five minutes are up, shake the basket around a bit and cook a few more minutes before serving.

Roasted Almonds

What's inside:

Paprika (1 tsp.)
Pepper (.25 tsp.)
Garlic powder (1 tbsp.)
Raw almonds (2 c.)
Soy sauce (1 tbsp.)

How to make:

1. Bring out a big bowl and add in all of the ingredients besides the almonds.

2. Stir them together so that you end up with a thick paste. Then add in the almonds so that they are coated with the paste.
3. Bring out an air fryer and turn it up to 320 degrees. Add the almonds and cook for a bit.
4. After 8 minutes have gone by, check out the almonds and see if they are done. Allow them some time to cool and then store or eat.

Vegan Meatballs

What's inside:

BBQ sauce (1.5 c.)
Whole berry cranberry sauce (1 can)
Vegan meatballs (2 lbs.)
Cornstarch with water (1 tbsp. each)
Water (.25 c.)

How to make:

1. Bring out the instant pot and add some water to it.
2. When the air fryer is hooked up, add the frozen vegan meatballs to this as well. Add in the cranberry sauce and BBQ and cover the meatballs with it.
3. Set this to a high pressure and seal it up. After five minutes, let the pressure come out naturally and remove the lid.
4. Add in the cornstarch and water mixture and stir around. Turn the pot back on to the saute setting and give the sauce a few minutes to thicken before serving.

Chapter 11: Week Four Meal Plan and Grocery List

Meal Plan

Day 1:	Day 2:	Day 3"	Day 4:
Breakfast: Apple Cinnamon Breakfast Lunch: Black Bean Burger Dinner: Pasta with tomatoes Snack: Chickpea Snack	Breakfast: Berry Smoothie Lunch: Vegan Pasta Puttanesca Dinner: Sweet Potato Quesadillas Snack: Fig Newtons	Breakfast: Breakfast Bowl Lunch: Vegan Tacos Dinner: Asian Baked Stuffed Sweet Potatoes Snack:	Breakfast: Sweet Potato Breakfast Bowl Lunch: Mexican Quinoa Dinner: Vegan Enchiladas Snack: Chickpea

		Vegan Snickers Bars	Snack
Day 5: Breakfast: Cajun Hash Browns Lunch: Black Bean Burger Dinner: Pasta with tomatoes Snack: Fig Newtons	Day 6 Breakfast: Berry Smoothie Lunch: Vegan Tacos Dinner: Sweet Potato Quesadilla Snack: Vegan Snickers Bars	Day 7: Breakfast: Breakfast Bowl Lunch: Mexican Quinoa Dinner: Vegan Enchiladas Snack: Fig Newtons	

Grocery List

6 corn tortillas	6 tortillas	6 whole wheat tortillas
2 c. chocolate chips	1 tbsp. vanilla	¾ c. coconut flour
¼ c. flax seed meal	3 tbsp. ground flax seed	1 handful coriander
¾ c. sugar	6 tbsp. nutritional yeast	2 ½ oats
1 can mixed beans	4 cans black beans	2 cans chickpeas
1 tbsp. capers	½ c. kalamata olives	4 c. pasta sauce
1 ½ c. applesauce	1 c. caramel sauce	2 tbsp. cashew butter
2 c. and 1 tbsp. almond butter	1 tbsp. peanut butter	1 can tomatoes
1 c. TVP	½ c. olive oil	1 c. salsa
2 c. red enchilada	¼ c. teriyaki sauce	2 tbsp. Sriracha sauce

sauce		
1 ½ c. almond milk	2 tbsp. Chili powder	3 tsp. cinnamon
2 tbsp. cumin	2 tsp. garlic powder	1 tsp. paprika
2 tbsp. smoked paprika	1 tsp. rosemary	Pepper
Salt	1 tsp. Cajun seasoning	1 tbsp. Taco seasoning
3 ½ c. quinoa	6 c. pasta	1 apple
1 avocado	2 banana	2 c. blueberries
1 c. corn	¼ c. edamame beans	3 garlic cloves
1 tbsp. minced onion	5 sweet potatoes	6 potatoes
2 handfuls spinach	1 can tomatoes	2 c. mixed vegetables
1 zucchini	2 packs tofu	3 c. dried figs
1 c. walnuts		

The Recipes

BREAKFAST

Apple Cinnamon Breakfast Cookies

What's inside:

Cinnamon (2 tsp.)
Diced apple (.5)
Applesauce (1.5 c.)
Sugar (.25 c.)
Old fashioned oats (2.5 c.)

How to make:

1. Turn on the oven and let it heat up to 350 degrees. Take out a baking sheet and prepare with some parchment paper.

2. Take out a bowl and mix the oats, cinnamon, and applesauce. Let this set for a bit and prepare your apple. Add the apple into this mixture.
3. Scoop this out and create some rounded mounds. Place these cookies onto the sheet and add into the oven.
4. After 20 minutes, the cookies will be done. Take them out of the oven and give them some time to cool before serving.

Berry Smoothie

What's inside:

Almond milk (.5 c.)
Almond butter (1 tbsp.)
Banana (1)
Water
Blueberries (1 c.)

How to make:

1. Take out a blender and add the almond milk blueberries, almond butter, and banana.
2. Add in the amount of water that is needed to thin out the smoothie to your preference.
3. Mix together well before serving.

Superfood Breakfast Bowl

What's inside:

Blueberries (.33 c.)
Almond milk (.33 c.)
Sliced banana (1)
Peanut butter (1 tbsp.)
Cooked quinoa (.5 c.)

How to make:

1. Cook the quinoa if it is not already done.
2. Bring out a bowl and then add all of the ingredients inside.
3. Serve this either warm or cold depending on your preference.

Sweet Potato Breakfast Bowl

What's inside

Cashew butter (2 tbsp.)
Cinnamon (.25 tsp.)
Almond milk (.25 c.)
Salt
Sweet potato, baked (1)

How to make:

1. Take all of the ingredients and blend them together using a food processor until smooth.

2. Use a rubber scraper to scrape this out of the food processor.
3. Add the toppings that you would like and then serve.

Cajun Hash Browns

What's inside:

Chili powder(1 tsp.)
Cajun seasoning (1 tsp.)
Paprika (1 tsp.)
Olive oil (.25 c.)
Potatoes, peeled (6)

How to make:

1. Start this recipe by heating the oven to 400 degrees. Add the potatoes to a baking sheet in a single layer.
2. Season with the Cajun spice, paprika, and chili. Drizzle on some olive oil.

3. Use a spatula to mix the potatoes around so that they are completely covered with the oil and the spices.
4. Add this to the oven and let it bake for a bit. After 40 minutes, the potatoes will be crisp and you can take them out and serve.

LUNCH

Black Bean Burger

What's inside

Cumin, ground (.5 tsp.)
Shredded zucchini (1)
Chili powder (1 tbsp.)
Ground flaxseed (3 tbsp.)
Salt (.5 tsp.)
Cooked black beans (2 c.)
Garlic powder (.5 tsp.)

How to make:

1. Drain and rinse the black beans. Put in half the black beans and flaxseed and mash them well.
2. Grate up the zucchini and squeeze off the extra water. Add into the mash

along with the black beans. Add seasoning and flaxseeds as well.
3. Take this to create six patties. Heat up some oil on a cast iron skillet and let it get nice and warm.
4. Add in the burgers and cook on medium heat. After six minutes, flip around and cook a bit longer.
5. Add your favorite toppings when you are ready to serve.

Vegan Pasta Puttanesca

What's inside:

Pepper
Salt
Water (3 c.)
Capers (1 tbsp.)
Pasta sauce (4 c.)
Sliced kalamata olives (.5 c.)
Minced garlic cloves (3)

Pasta (4 c.)

How to make:

1. Bring out the Instant Pot and add a bit of water and the garlic. Cook for half a minute. Turn the pot off and add in the capers, water, olives, pasta, and pasta sauce.
2. Mix these all together and then seal on the lead of the air fryer. Set the timer on manual for a bit.
3. After five minutes, use the quick release pressure and then open the lid. Add some pepper and salt and then serve.

Vegan Tacos

What's inside:

Corn tortillas (6)
Salt
Drained black beans (1 can)

TVP (1 c.)

Dried minced onions (.5 tbsp.)

Taco seasoning (1 tbsp.)

Water (.75 c.)

Toppings of choice

How to make:

1. Take out a pot and add in the taco seasoning, onion, and water. Bring all of this to a boil.
2. When this reaches boiling, add in the TVP and put on low heat. Let it absorb the liquid.
3. Add in the beans and the lid on top. Cook for a few minutes until they are done.
4. Heat up the tortillas in a pan with some oil until they are nice and crispy. Take the filling from the heat and put it into the tortillas.

5. Put on the toppings of your choice and serve.

Mexican Quinoa

What's inside:

Cilantro
Black beans (1 can)
Ground cumin (1 tbsp.)
Corn kernels (1 c.)
Jarred salsa (1 c.)
Cooked white quinoa (3 c.)

How to make:

1. Take out a large skillet and heat it up. Add in the corn and black beans and cook to make the corn tender.
2. Add in the quinoa and stir. Cook for a bit longer to make the quinoa hot before adding in the salsa.

3. After another two minutes, take the skillet off the heat and give it time to cool down.
4. Fluff up the quinoa with a fork and serve.

DINNER

Pasta with Tomatoes and Beans

What's inside:

Oil (1 tbsp.)
Salt (1 tsp.)
Pasta (2 c.)
Spinach (2 handfuls)
Cherry tomatoes (1 can)
Mixed beans (1 can)
Crushed tomatoes (1 can)

How to make

1. Follow the directions on the package to cook up the pasta. Open up the beans and rinse them off.

2. Add a bit of oil to the pan and heat it up. Add in the beans and crushed tomatoes. Bring to a gentle boil.
3. Take the cherry tomatoes and slice in half before adding them to the pan. Cook for a bit longer.
4. Add in the spinach and salt and turn down the heat. Stir and cook a few more minutes and then serve.

Sweet Potato Quesadillas

What's inside

Sriracha sauce (2 tbsp.)
Tortillas (6)
Salt
Smoked paprika (2 tbsp.)
Nutritional yeast (6 tbsp.)
Steamed sweet potatoes (2 c.)

How to make:

1. Bring out a bowl and add in the salt, yeast, paprika, Sriracha sauce, and sweet potatoes.
2. Take a fork and use it to mash up the ingredients in the bowl. A food processor can be used as well.
3. Spread this onto 4 tortillas and then cover with another tortilla.
4. Add to a skillet and toast on both sides and enjoy.

Asian Baked Stuffed Sweet Potatoes

What's inside

Coriander and sesame seeds (1 handful)
Vegetables of choice
Shelled edamame beans (.25 c.)
Teriyaki sauce (.25 c.)
Tofu (200 grams)

Sweet potatoes (2)

How to make:

1. Turn the oven on to 200 degrees. Take your sweet potatoes and slice them lengthwise.
2. Wrap in some foil and add to the oven to bake for 45 minutes. As this is cooking, slice up the tofu and add to a bowl.
3. Pour in the teriyaki sauce and cover the cubes up. Prepare the other vegetables that you chose.
4. Take the potatoes out and scoop out the middle. Fill up the potato with the tofu and the vegetables and place back into the oven.
5. Bring out a baking bowl and fill with water. Add the edamame beans and place in the oven.

6. After 15 more minutes, the beans and potatoes are done and you can take them out.

Vegan Enchiladas

What's inside:

Avocado (1)
Canned black beans (2 c.)
Red enchilada sauce (2 c.)
Organic tofu (1 pack)
Whole wheat vegan tortillas (6)

How to make

1. Turn on the oven to 350 degrees. Take the tofu and slice into cubes.
2. Add some oil to a skillet and stir fry the tofu, adding in some of the seasonings of your choice.

3. Lay out the tortillas and fill them with the beans, tofu cubes, and half the sauce. Roll these up.
4. Take out a casserole dish and add the tortillas inside. Top the enchiladas with the sauce and add to the oven.
5. After 20 minutes, the dish is done. Top with avocado and enjoy.

SNACK

Fig Newtons

What's inside:

Flaxseed meal (.25 c.)
Vanilla (1 tbsp.)
Walnut halves (1 c.)
Salt (.5 tsp.)
Dried figs (3 c.)

How to make:

1. Take out your food processor and place all of the ingredients inside.
2. Turn the food processor on and let it pulse for a bit to make a sand-like mixture.
3. Take the blade from the food processor and place it to the side. Scoop out the

mixture to make little balls with the help of an ice cream scoop.
4. Roll this mixture using your hands to make more of these balls. You can add them into a container and leave in the fridge for up to seven days when done.

Chickpea Snack

What's inside:

Garlic powder (1.5 tsp.)
Ground rosemary (1 tsp.)
Olive oil (1.5 tbsp.)
Pepper
Salt
Drained chickpeas (2 cans)

How to make:

1. Turn on the oven and let it heat up to 375 degrees. While that is warming up,

take out a baking sheet and line with some parchment paper.
2. Drain out the chickpeas and rinse them off. Dry them well using some kitchen towels.
3. Add the chickpeas to a baking sheet with the rosemary as well. Then place the baking sheet into the oven to bake.
4. After 15 minutes, the chickpeas should be done and you can take them out of the oven.
5. Bring out a bowl and add in the toasted chickpeas along with the nutmeg, olive oil, pepper, salt, and garlic powder.
6. Put these back on the baking sheet and back into the oven.
7. After 20 more minutes, take everything out of the oven and give it some time to cool down before serving.

Vegan Snickers Bars

What's inside:

Sticky Sweetener (.5 c.)
Water (2 tbsp)
Almond butter (2 c.)
Keto caramel sauce (1 serving)
Coconut flour (.75 c.)
Chocolate chips (2 c.)

How to make:

1. Bring out a bowl and add the coconut flour inside. Set to the side.
2. Add the sweetener and almond butter to a bowl and combine. Melt in the microwave until well combined.
3. Add this to the coconut flour to make a batter. Add this to a baking dish that is prepared and press down firmly. Place in the fridge.

4. Prepare the caramel sauce and then add into the baking dish. Place in the fridge until it firms up.
5. Melt the chocolate chips and pour over the dish. Put into the fridge for another half hour before serving.

Chapter 12: Week Five Meal Plan and Grocery List

MEAL PLAN

Day 1:	Day 2:	Day 3:	Day 4:
Breakfast: Ginger Plums	Breakfast: Walnut Porridge	Breakfast: Coconut Cream Berry Bowl	Breakfast: Raspberry Chia Pudding
Lunch: Avocado Zucchini Noodles	Lunch: Summer Pasta	Lunch: Bibimbap	Lunch Zucchini Lasagna
Dinner: Jackfruit Taco Bowls	Dinner: Gnocchi and Broccoli Bake	Dinner: Avocado and Hummus Quesadillas	Dinner: Spicy Garlic Pasta
Snack: Chocolate Coconut Bars	Snacks: Coconut milk Ice	Snack: Quinoa Fudge	Snack: Chocolate Coconut Bars

	Cream		
Day 5:	Day 6:	Day 7:	
Breakfast: Bagel Thins Lunch: Avocado Zucchini Noodles Dinner: Jackfruit Taco Bowls Snack: Coconut Milk ice cream	Breakfast: Walnut Porridge Lunch: Summer Pasta Dinner: Gnocchi and Broccoli Bake Snack: Quinoa Fudge	Breakfast: Ginger Plums Lunch Zucchini Lasagna Dinner: Spicy Garlic Pasta Snack: Chocolate Coconut Bars	

GROCERY LIST

2 tortillas	1 tsp. baking powder	½ c. chocolate chips
2 tbsp. cocoa powder	5 tsp. vanilla	1 vanilla pod
2 tbsp. and ½ c. chia seeds	3 tbsp. flaxseed	2 tbsp. hemp seed
1 tbsp. sesame seeds	1 ½ tbsp. cornstarch	½ c. sugar
3 tbsp. maple syrup	2 tbsp. nutritional yeast	2 tbsp. hummus
25 oz. marinara sauce	½ c. and 2 tbsp. coconut cream	4 can coconut milk
½ c. Tahini	¼ c. sun dried tomatoes	2 c. vegan cheese
3 tbsp. coconut oil	6 tbsp. olive oil	¾ c. almond milk
1 c. frozen kale	1 ¼ c. basil	1 tp. Red chili flakes

½ tsp. cinnamon	2 pieces ginger	5 mint leaves
Salt	Pepper	2 tbsp. taco seasoning
½ c. quinoa	2 c. fettuccini pasta	10 oz. pasta
2 packages cauliflower rice	2 avocados	4 c. berries
4 c. broccoli	1 carrot	10 oz. riced cauliflower
2 ½ c. coconut	½ cucumber	10 garlic cloves
5 tbsp. lemon juice	1 orange	1 c. peas
1 red bell pepper	5 plums	1 c. raspberries
12 cherry tomatoes	1 c. cherry tomatoes	3 zucchini
7 oz. tempeh	14 oz. firm tofu	8 Medjool dates
4 Tbsp. pine nuts	1 ½ c. walnuts	1 tsp. birch xylitol
½ c. psyllium husk powder	2 tbsp Sriracha	1 can young jackfruit

THE RECIPES

BREAKFAST

Ginger Plums

What's inside:

Water (5 tbsp.)
Cinnamon (.5 tsp.)
Zest of one orange
Pitted and sliced plums (5)
Ginger (2 pieces)

How to make

1. Turn on the oven to 375. Place the plums onto a baking tray with the flesh down.

2. Mix the cinnamon, water, ginger, and orange zest together and then pour over the plums.
3. Add to the oven and bake. After 20 minutes, take them out of the oven and give them time to cool before serving.

Walnut Porridge

What's inside:

Hemp seeds (2 tbsp.)
Chopped walnuts (.5 c.)
Whole chia seeds (2 tbsp.)
Almond milk (.75 c.)
Coconut milk (.25 c.)

How to make

1. Take out a pan and pour in the coconut and almond milk. Stir this and let it warm up.

2. When warm, take off the heat and combine inside the hemp seeds, chia seeds, and walnuts.
3. Stir to combine and set aside.
4. After 10 minutes, scoop this into your serving bowls and top with some toasted coconut before serving.

Coconut Cream Berry Bowl

What's inside:

Birch xylitol (1 tsp.)
Chilled coconut milk (1 can)
Vanilla pod (1)
Berries of choice (4 c.)
Minced mint leaves (5 pieces)

How to make:

1. Cut up the berries into small pieces and then add to a mixing bowl. Add the

minced leaves in as well and toss to combine.
2. Scoop out the solidified coconut milk and place into a bowl. Get rid of the coconut liquid. Cut the ends of the vanilla pod and scrape out the seeds. Add to the coconut cream.
3. Beat the seeds with the cream until well mixed. Add in the xylitol and mix to make nice and fluffy.
4. Top with the berries and add some fresh mint to this as well before serving.

Raspberry Chia Pudding

What's inside:

Vanilla (3 tsp.)
Raspberries (1 c.)
Whole chia seeds (.5 c.)
Coconut milk (1 c.)
Water (.5 c.)

How to make:

1. Take out a blender and mix together the coconut milk, water, and raspberries. Blend together well.
2. Combine the raspberry milk, chia seeds, vanilla, and stevia if you choose into a bowl.
3. Put into the fridge for half an hour. When ready, scoop into some serving glasses and top with raspberries before serving.

Bagel Thins

What's inside:

Sesame seeds
Baking powder (1 tsp.)
Salt

Psyllium husk powder (.5 c.)

Ground flaxseed (3 tbsp.)

Tahini (.5 c.)

How to make:

1. Heat up the oven to 375 degrees. Take out a bowl and whisk together the husk powder, flax seeds, baking powder, and salt.
2. Add in a cup of water to combine a bit and then the tahini.
3. Shape this into small patties and place onto a baking tray. Make sure to poke a small hole into each one.
4. Top with sesame seeds and then add to the oven to bake. After 40 minutes, take these out to cool. Cut into each one like a bagel and then serve.

LUNCH

Avocado Zucchini Noodles

What's inside:

Sliced cherry tomatoes (12)
Avocado (1)
Lemon juice (2 tbsp.)
Pine nuts (4 tbsp.)
Water (.33 c.)
Basil (1.25 c.)
Zucchini (1)

How to make

1. Use a peeler to make the zucchini into noodles.
2. Take out a blender and add in all of the ingredients besides the tomatoes inside. Blend to make them smooth.

3. Bring out a mixing bowl and add in the cherry tomatoes, avocados, and zucchini noodles. Serve!

Summer Pasta

What's inside:

Pepper (.25 tsp.)
Salt (.25 tsp.)
Olive oil (3 tbsp.)
Cherry tomatoes (1 c.)
Peas (1 .)
Salt (.5 tsp.)
Pasta (10 oz.)

How to make:

1. Boil some water in a skillet. Add in some salt and some oil. Boil the pasta inside.
2. After 7 minutes, drain out the pasta, but leave a bit of water. In the same skillet,

boil some more water and cook the peas for a bit.

3. Drain out the water and add the peas to some cold water.
4. Heat up some oil in a skillet and add the tomatoes. Let these cook so they become tender. Add in the pepper and salt to finish.
5. Now add in the rest of the water, the peas, and the pasta. Stir around and then serve.

Bibimbap

What's inside

Riced cauliflower (10 oz.)
Sriracha (2 tbsp.)
Grated carrot (1)
Julienned cucumber (.5)
Julienned red bell pepper (1)
Sliced broccoli (4)

Sliced tempeh (7 oz.)

How to make

1. Bring out a bowl and combine the vinegar and soy sauce. Immerse the tempeh into this for a few minutes.
2. Bring out a skillet and heat up the oil inside. Fry the tempeh and remove when it turns brown.
3. In the same skillet, cook the peppers, broccoli, and carrots. When they are done, set to the side.
4. Bring out another pan and heat up the oil. Toss in the cauliflower and cook until soft. Add in the chili paste and soy sauce.
5. Portion the riced cauliflower into bowls and add in the tempeh, vegetables, and cucumbers.
6. Top with some chili sauce and serve.

Zucchini Lasagna

What's inside:

Chopped sun-dried tomatoes (.25 c.)
Marinara sauce (25 oz.)
Ground walnuts (1 c.)
Lasagna
Pepper
Salt
Lemon juice (1 tbsp.)
Firm tofu (14 oz.)
Nutritional yeast (2 tbsp.)
Zucchini (2)

How to make:

1. Turn on the oven to 375 degrees. Take out your food processor and mix together the olive oil, lemon juice, and tofu inside.

2. In another bowl, mix together the tomatoes, sauce, and walnuts.
3. Slice up the zucchini going the long way. Take out a baking pan and add the marinara sauce on the bottom. Add the noodles and then spread 1/3 of the tofu over it all. Sprinkle on the nutritional yeast and the walnut sauce.
4. Layer back and forth until all of the ingredients are gone. Place into the oven to bake.
5. After 35 minutes, this is done and you can serve.

DINNER

Jackfruit and Cauliflower Taco Bowls

What's inside

Vegan cheese for serving
Olive oil (1 tbsp.)
Cauliflower rice (2 packages)
Frozen kale (1 c.)
Taco seasoning (2 tbsp.)
Young Jackfruit (1 can)

How to make

1. Chop the jackfruit into smaller sizes. Add everything but the cheese to the pot.
2. Cook these all together until the cauliflower has time to become nice and tender.

3. When ready, serve with some vegan cheese and guacamole if you would like.

Gnocchi and Broccoli Bake

What's inside:

Pepper
Salt
Vegan cheese (1 c.)
Tomato sauce (1 jar)
Cannellini beans (1 can)
Gnocchi (1 package)
Broccoli florets (4 c.)

How to make

1. Turn on the oven and let it heat up to 400 degrees. While this is heating up, boil some water and cook the broccoli for two minutes.

2. Add in the gnocchi and cook. After 5 minutes drain out the water and put the gnocchi and broccoli back in the pot.
3. Add .75 cup of cheese, tomato sauce, and cannellini beans to this. Mix and then pour into a baking dish.
4. Spread these ingredients out and top with the rest of the cheese. Add to the oven to bake.
5. After 20 minutes, the dish will be done. Take out of the oven and serve.

Avocado and Hummus Quesadillas

What's inside:

Pepper
Salt
Vegan cheese
Hummus (2 tbsp.)
Sliced avocado (1)
Tortillas (2)

How to make

1. Use a cookie cutter to make small tortillas out of the big one.
2. Take each tortilla and spread the hummus on one side. Add on some avocado and sprinkle with cheese.
3. Fold these tortillas up and cook on a skillet for a few minutes before serving.

Spicy Garlic Pasta

What's inside:

Olive oil (2 tbsp.)
Garlic (10 cloves)
Red chili flakes (1 tsp.)
Lemon juice (1.5 tbsp.)
Fettuccini pasta (200 g.)

How to make:

1. Take the fettuccine pasta and cook by following the directions on the package.
2. While this is cooking, chop up the garlic cloves and squeeze the lemon to take out the juice.
3. Place the cooked pasta in some cold water and set to the side.
4. Heat up some oil in a skillet and cook the garlic for a minute. Add in the chili flakes to warm up.
5. Add the pasta to the pan and the lemon juice. Heat for a minute before serving.

SNACKS

Chocolate Coconut Bars

What's inside:

Coconut bars
Coconut oil, melted (2 tbsp.)
Coconut cream (.25 c. and 2 tbsp)
Pure maple syrup (3 tbsp.)
Coconut unsweetened (2.5 c.)
Chocolate layer
Vegan chocolate chips(.5 c.)
Coconut cream (.25 c.)

How to make

1. Prepare a baking dish with some parchment paper. Then add the ingredients for the coconut mixture to a

food processor. Mix to get a nice sticky mixture.
2. Add this to the baking pan and press down into a smooth layer.
3. To make the chocolate layer, add the chocolate chips and coconut cream to a double broiler until they are melted.
4. Pour this over the coconut mixture and spread it out. Add to the freezer.
5. After an hour, slice up and enjoy.

Coconut Milk Ice Cream

What's inside

Cornstarch (1.5 tbsp.)
Salt (.25 tsp.)
Sugar (.5 c.)
Vanilla (2 tsp.)
Coconut milk (2 cans)

How to make:

1. Take out half a cup of coconut milk and set to the side. Put the rest in a pan with the salt and sugar and whisk to dissolve.
2. Add the cornstarch to the reserved coconut milk and then bring to a boil with the other ingredients.
3. After 5 minutes of boiling and stirring, it should thicken. Put this into a shallow container and leave in the fridge for a bit.
4. After four hours, put this into a frozen ice cream bowl and start to churn, using the instructions on your machine.
5. Serve when it reaches the desired consistency.

Quinoa Fudge

What's inside:

Flaked sea salt
Cocoa powder (2 tbsp.)
Melted coconut oil (1 tbsp.)
Medjool dates (8)
Water (3 tbsp.)
Uncooked quinoa (.5 c.)

How to make:

1. Toast the quinoa in a dry skillet for a few minutes. Then add to a blender to turn into a flour mixture.
2. Add the quinoa with the dates, coconut oil, and cocoa powder until they combine. Add in a bit of water at a time to make a dough.
3. Take out a sandwich-sized container and line with plastic wrap. Add the

dough to this container and press it down to make smooth.
4. Put into the fridge to set. This can take three hours or more. When done, slice into small pieces and serve.

Chapter 13: Week Six Meal Plan and Grocery List

THE MEAL PLAN

Day 1	Day 2	Day 3:	Day 4:
Breakfast: Vegan Protein Shake Lunch: Coconut Curry Dinner: Vegan Pizza Snack: Almond Cookies	Breakfast: Tofu Veggie Scramble Lunch: Italian Potato Curry Dinner: Vegan Pita Snack: Sweet Potato Brownies	Breakfast: Flaxseed Waffles Lunch: Easy Tofu Bake Dinner: Hummus Pasta Snack: Sweet Potato Brownies	Breakfast: Eggplant Hole Lunch: Tofu Vegetable Curry Dinner: Creamy Kale Pasta Snack: Mince Pies
Day 5:	Day 6:	Day 7:	

Breakfast: Vegan Protein Shake Lunch: Italian Potato Curry Dinner: Vegan Pizza Snack: Almond Cookies	Breakfast: Tofu Veggie Scramble Lunch: Easy Tofu Bake Dinner: Hummus Pasta Snack: Mince Pies	Breakfast: Flaxseed Waffles Lunch: Coconut Curry Dinner: Vegan Pita Snack: Almond Cookies	

THE GROCERY LIST

2 pita breads	1 tbsp. baking powder	½ sp. Vanilla
2 c. flour	¾ c. almond meal	2 c. golden flaxseed
1 tbsp. cornstarch	1 c. golden caster sugar	1 tbsp. maple syrup
¾ c. oats	1 can chickpeas	½ c. hummus
¾ c. garlic hummus	2 Tbsp. red curry paste	5 cans coconut milk
2 tbsp. almond butter	½ c. coconut oil	1 tbsp. sesame oil
1 c. olive oil	4 tbsp. green curry paste	1 tbsp. garlic paste
½ tsp. hot pepper sauce	3 tbsp. tamari	1 tsp. butter
120 g. dairy free margarine	9 flax eggs	½ c. almond milk
1/3 c. non-dairy milk	1 tbsp. red chili powder	1 tbsp. ground cinnamon

½ tbsp. cumin powder	1 bunch coriander	¼ c. parsley
Salt	½ tsp. turmeric powder	½ c. hemp hearts
300 g. mince meat	16 oz. pasta	1 handful arugula
1 avocado	1 banana	5 c. broccoli
1 eggplant	6 garlic cloves	½ c. garlic
4 c. kale	1 tbsp. lemon juice	1 c. mushrooms
¼ red onion	2 sweet potatoes	3 potatoes
2 green onions	10 bunches spinach	1 c. cherry tomatoes
3 tomatoes	¾ zucchini	1 pizza dough
3 ½ lbs. tofu	225 g dark chocolate	1 c. packed dates
1 c. cashews	1 tbsp. chia seeds	

THE RECIPES

BREAKFAST

Vegan Protein Shake

What's inside:

Salt
Vanilla (.5 tsp.)
Hemp hearts (.5 c.)
Chia seeds (1 tbsp.)
Coconut milk (.66 c.)

How to make:

1. Add all of the ingredients into a container and shut the lid tightly.
2. Stir and combine.

3. Chill this overnight. The next day, take it out of the container and then add in the milk before serving.

Tofu Veggie Scramble

What's inside:

Firm tofu (2 lbs.)
Spinach (10 bunches)
Sliced mushrooms (1 c.)
Minced garlic cloves (4)
Chopped tomatoes (3)
Olive oil (3 tbsp.)

How to make:

1. Heat up some oil in a skillet and cook the mushrooms, garlic, and tomatoes together.

2. After three minutes, reduce the heat and add in the lemon juice, soy sauce, tofu, and spinach. Continue to cook.
3. After another 7 minutes, take this off the heat and serve warm.

Flaxseed Waffles

What's inside:

Golden flaxseed (2 c.)
Melted coconut oil (.33 c.)
Ground cinnamon (1 tbsp.)
Flax eggs (5)
Baking powder (1 tbsp.)

How to make:

1. Turn on the waffle iron. Then prepare the flax eggs by combining the flax meal with water and setting aside.

2. Add the salt, flax seed, and baking powder into a bowl and whisk well. Add in the oil, the flax eggs, and half a cup of water to a blender and mix together well.
3. Move this to a bowl and stir to make fluffy. Add in the cinnamon.
4. Scoop a portion of this batter into the waffle machine and cook until they are done. Repeat until the batter is gone.

Eggplant Hole

What's inside

Green onion stalks (2)
Eggs (4)
Butter (1 tsp.)
Olive oil (1 tbsp.)
Eggplant (1)

How to make

1. Turn on your grill to heat up. Then take the eggplant and cut into slices. Brush with olive oil and sprinkle on the pepper and salt.
2. Add this to the grill and cook on each side for a few minutes.
3. Cut a hole in the middle of each and then cook on a heated pan. Add the egg mixture to the middle of each eggplant.
4. Give the egg time to cook and then serve with some sliced green onions and enjoy.

LUNCH

Coconut Curry

What's inside:

Garlic, minced
Cornstarch (1 tbsp.)
Chickpeas (1 can)
Broccoli heads (2)
Red curry paste (2 tbsp.)
Coconut milk (1 can)

How to make:

1. Start out by adding some oil to a pan and heating up. Then cook the garlic and broccoli together for a few minutes.
2. Add in the coconut milk and let it simmer. After 8 minutes, add in the curry paste and whisk to combine.

3. Add in the chickpeas and bring this to a boil before adding in the cornstarch.
4. After another minute of boiling, reduce the heat and allow the sauce to thicken as things cool. Serve warm.

Indian Potato Curry

What's inside

Cooking oil (3 tbsp.)
Salt
Coriander (1 bunch)
Turmeric powder (.5 tsp.)
Cumin powder (.5 tbsp.)
Red chili powder (1 tbsp.)
Garlic paste (1 Tbsp.)
Potatoes (3)
Water (2 c.)

How to make

1. Peel and cube the potatoes. Take out a pan and add in the oil and garlic to heat up for half a minute.
2. Add in the potato cubes and cook for two more minutes before adding in all of your spices.
3. After a few seconds of mixing, add in the water, making sure it is enough to cover the potatoes.
4. After 20 minutes of cooking, the potatoes will be done. When the sauce is thick, add in some coriander and cook a bit longer before serving.

Easy Tofu Bake

What's inside:

Hot pepper sauce (.5 tsp.)
Sesame oil (1 tbsp.)

Maple syrup (1 tbsp.)

Tamari (3 tbsp.)

Tofu (8 oz.)

How to make

1. Turn on the oven to 400 degrees. While that is warming up, bring out a baking dish and spray with some cooking spray.
2. Drain out the tofu. Wrap into a towel and press for 15 minutes to drain it out. Then slice into two pieces. Cut each part into 16 pieces.
3. Bring out a bowl and combine the rest of the ingredients to make your marinade. Pour this over the tofu. Let it set.
4. After 30 minutes, drain the tofu and then place these on a baking sheet. Add to the oven.
5. After 10 minutes, take the dish out, turn everything over, and bake again. In 12 minutes, the pieces will be done.Give

them time to cool before serving.

Tofu Vegetable Curry

What's inside:

Coconut milk (3 cans)
Green vegan curry paste (4 tbsp.)
Sweet potatoes (2)
Salt
Olive oil
Firm tofu (12 oz.)
Broccoli (3 c.)

How to make:

1. Take out the tofu and drain it out before slicing into cubes.
2. Heat up some oil in a pot and then add in the tofu. Fry the tofu for a bit until they turn golden brown.
3. Take out another pot and add in the vegan curry paste, coconut milk, and sweet potatoes. Simmer these for a bit.

4. After 10 minutes, add in the broccoli and cook for a few more minutes to get those done before serving.

DINNER

Vegan Pizza with Avocado

What's inside:

Crushed pepper flakes
Salt
Olive oil
Arugula (1 handful)
Avocado (1)
Pizza dough (1)

How to make:

1. Turn on the oven and let it heat up to 500 degrees.
2. Roll out the pizza dough and place the dough on a baking steel in the oven. After three minutes, rotate the pizza so

it is evenly baked. Bake for another two minutes.
3. During this time, peel and crush the avocados. Take the pizza out of the oven and spread the avocados on top.
4. Add the arugula and drizzle on the olive oil, salt, and red pepper flakes before serving.

Vegan Pita Pizza

What's inside:

Cherry tomatoes (.5 pint)
Red onion (.25)
Zucchini (.75)
Chipotle hummus (as needed)
Pita bread (2)

How to make:

1. Turn on the oven and let it heat up to 425 degrees. Bring out a baking sheet and add parchment paper.
2. Place the pita onto this sheet and then spread out the chipotle on each one.
3. Sprinkle the cherry tomatoes, red onion, and zucchini on top. Add to the oven and let it bake.
4. After 10 minutes, the pizza is done. Takeout of the oven and serve warm.

Hummus Pasta

What's inside

Pepper
Salt
Parsley (.25 c.)
Non-dairy milk (.33 c.)
Cherry tomatoes (.5 c.)
Garlic hummus (.75 c.)
Pasta (8 oz.)

How to make:

1. Follow the directions on the package to make the pasta. When it is done, drain out the water and put into the pot again.
2. Add the ingredients to the pot and mix well. Adjust the spices as needed.
3. Divide into four bowls and enjoy.

Creamy Kale Pasta

What's inside:

Salt
Garlic (2 cloves)
Olive oil (1 tbsp.)
Kale (4 c.)
For the sauce
Almond milk (.5 c.)
Cashews (1 c.)
Lemon juice
Olive oil (.25 c.)

Salt (1 tsp.)

Garlic (.25 c.)

Pasta (8 oz.)

How to make:

1. Soak the cashews in some water for two hours. Drain and rinse them after this time.
2. Heat up some oil in a pan and then add in the garlic and kale. Cook these until they become soft.
3. During this time, add in the sauce ingredients to a blender and mix to make smooth.
4. Cook the pasta by following the directions on the package. Drain out the water, but save it for later.
5. Mix the pasta with the water, kale, and sauce before serving.

SNACKS

Almond Cookies

What's inside:

Gluten-free rolled oats (.75 c.)
Almond meal .75 c.)
Almond butter (2 tbsp.)
Banana (1)
Packed dates (1 c.)

How to make

1. Add the dates to your food processor and turn them into small bits.
2. Add in the banana and almond butter and pulse to combine. Add in the almond meal and the oats.

3. Add to a bowl and add in some almond meal if it is too sticky. Let it chill in the fridge for a bit.
4. During that time, turn on the oven to 350 degrees and give it time to heat up.
5. Scoop the dough onto a baking tray and then add to the oven. After 15 minutes, take it out and give it time to cool before serving.

Sweet Potato Brownies

What's inside:

Oats (.5 c.)
Cocoa powder (10 tbsp.)
Raw almonds (.5 c.)
Coconut sugar (6 tbsp.)
Sweet potatoes (1 lb.)

How to make:

1. Turn on the oven to 355 degrees. Peel and chop the sweet potato. Steam for 25 minutes to make soft.
2. Add the almonds to a food processor and pulse to get almond flour. Add in the ingredients and pulse well, including sweet potato.
3. Add this to your baking dish and then to the oven. After 30 minutes, the brownies will be done.

Mince Pies

What's inside:

Golden caster sugar (150g)
Plain flour (2 c.)
Mincemeat (300 g.)
Dairy-free margarine (120 g.)
Dairy-free dark chocolate (225 g)

How to make:

1. Turn on the oven to 320 degrees. Prepare a baking tin with some parchment paper.
2. Take out a bowl and add in the chocolate and butter. Add an inch of water to a pan and let it simmer. Add the bowl on top.
3. Stir these ingredients on occasion, waiting for them to melt completely. Take off the heat when it is done and stir together the mincemeat, sugar, and flour in as well.
4. Add this to your prepared baking tin and press down. Add to the oven to bake.
5. After 45 minutes, take the dish out. Give them some time to cool down before serving.

Conclusion

Thank for making it through to the end of *Vegan Diet Meal Planning*. Let's hope it was informative and able to provide you with all of the tools you need to achieve your goals, whatever they may be.

The next step is to get started on this diet plan. We have spent some time talking about the vegan diet, and how you can combine that with meal planning to really make your life easier. With the tips and the techniques that we have expressed in this guidebook, and all of the great recipes and meal plans for the first six weeks, you will be able to get started on this diet plan and fit it into your life, no matter how busy you are.

If you have been interested in the vegan diet in the past and are ready to get started with it, but you just weren't ready to fit it into that busy schedule, then this guidebook is the right option for you. Check it out and see exactly how you can add meal planning to the vegan diet to improve your health and help you to see the best results.

Finally, if you found this book useful in anyway, a review on Amazon is always appreciated!

www.ingramcontent.com/pod-product-compliance
Lightning Source LLC
Chambersburg PA
CBHW071231070526
44583CB00017B/2132